The Unexpected Journey

Hennie Friedman

DEDICATIONS

I dedicate this book to the three Angels that have cared and continue to care for my husband as though he were a beloved relative:

Norma Pringle—who has a heart of gold.
Guylene Monpleisor—who is gentle and sensitive.
Kim Lovell—who has loads of energy and a smile that lights up the room.

I also dedicate this book to **Malka Fass**, who fights bureaucracy to ensure that Moish and many others like him has the best care possible. Malka is a beautiful person who personifies kindness and does so much for others in the most humble and unassuming way.

My love and gratitude to my amazing children (all 16) and grandchildren, who are my anchors and the joy of my life.

Thank you **Perele** for all your love and all your help.

Hertzie and **Lolly**: Thank you for constantly checking up on me, for never giving up on me, and for helping me out financially through tough times.

To all my nieces and nephews—I love you all. Extra hugs for the special few that spent so much time with my mom during the last eight years of her life, enabling me to have more time and energy for my husband. (I believe that your father, my brother, may he rest in peace, is smiling down on you.)

To my amazing *machatonim* (parents of my in-law children) and to all my beloved friends—you know who you are!! I love you so much!!

To my "adopted children" for being such a special part of my life.

To the staff and children at HASC (past and present), I have been privileged to work with you over the last 30 years!

Thank you Jim Gratiot for helping me take my dream and make it a reality.

Most important, of course: thank you to *Hashem* for giving me the opportunity to write this memoir.

PROLOGUE

Far Rockaway, New York
February 21, 2018

Eighteen months ago, my beautiful husband frequently lost his smile.

Moish now spends his days and nights in a large, comfortable hospital bed that faces the framed wedding portraits of all eight of our children. There are other pictures in his bedroom as well — one of Moish and his granddaughter smiling at Chuck E. Cheese's; one of Moish cutting the cake at one of our children's birthday parties; and one of Moish and I looking young and happy during the three years we lived in Israel.

Moish is surrounded by pictures of his family and friends—but we don't know if he recognizes them.

Outside his fifth-story window is a spectacular view of the beach and the ocean. We moved to this condominium in Far Rockaway two years ago to be closer to four of our children. Two others live a couple of hours away, while still two others live in Chicago and Florida.

Moish does not seem to know the names of his children or grandchildren, although he still responds to his name and seems to recognize me and some of our kids. Moish lies in bed most of the day with a neatly trimmed beard and drool on his chin. His eyes are sometimes lifeless and his smile, which used to light up the whole room, is rarely seen. Occasionally—and sometimes appropriately—he will flash a beautiful smile.

Moish is seldom alone, as he has three aides who take care of him around the clock. Today, one of his aides, Norma, sits in a rocking chair and talks quietly to him; she has been with Moish the longest, nearly ten years. She likes to tell him funny stories about her day. Several times a week, weather permitting, Norma takes Moish out for an afternoon walk in his wheelchair. They stroll along the beach, a jaunty hat shielding his eyes from the reflection of the sun off the water.

Sometimes I excuse Norma or the other aides early so I can spend time alone with my husband. Just the two of us, like the old days... except that now I am in a permanent state of exhaustion. It comforts me, in some odd way, to hold Moish's hand and tell him about our kids and our grandkids. I tell him about my day at work, or reminisce about some of the crazy adventures we had when we were young. It's during these talks that I think about the life Moish and I had together, and about the dreams that will never come to pass.

I try to be optimistic when I'm with Moish. Sometimes I sing to him, or play him television shows we used to watch or songs we used to dance to. Sometimes I lie next to him and cry, wishing that just once more he would give me a kiss or speak my name.

My mind wanders occasionally during my times alone with Moish. I think about errands I have to run, or about paperwork that I have to do the next day at work, or about a funny story my daughter told me over the phone. Other times my mind is deadly focused, thinking about the glorious times before Moish got sick, or about the confusing times when he first showed signs of this terrible disease.

Mostly, though, I think about the times when Moish still knew how to smile.

CHAPTER 1

On our first date, in the early Seventies, Moish escorted me to the Café Feenjon, a loud, vibrant café in Greenwich Village that featured live Greek-Israeli music and an assortment of exotic drinks. I was eighteen years old at the time, attending the Beth Israel School of Nursing in Manhattan. Moish was five years older than I was, but my mother had instilled in me the belief that women were more mature than men, so our age difference didn't bother me. I sat across the table from him, music thumping in my ears, nervously admiring his wonderful smile. When Moish smiled, he made me feel like I was the only girl in the room.

Three of our mutual friends had set us up, each of them insisting that Moish was funny and generous and handsome—in other words, a great catch! My first impression was that he was the opposite of what I was looking for. I was searching for the traditional tall, dark, and handsome stranger—a modern-day Valentino—whereas Moish was petite, thin, and cute. He was only one inch taller than me, and not physically strong. Two years later, when I lovingly asked him to carry me over the hotel threshold after our wedding, he looked like he was going to have a hernia.

Then there was his job. I had always envisioned myself marrying somebody with a glamorous career—a doctor, a corporate lawyer, a college professor. Moish told me he was an accountant, a job I associated with thick black glasses and a slide rule in the pocket of his starched white shirt. The interesting thing was that Moish didn't do any actual accounting when I met him. Instead, he helped his father run a hotel in Long Beach for elderly tenants. Moish worked at that job for only seven months, walking away when he realized it wasn't in his best interest, emotionally speaking, to work with his family, even though he was very close to them.

According to the friends who set us up, Moish had dated many girls before me, and must have frequented the Café Feenjon often. Moish was even close with the manager—they greeted each other like brothers, and it was the manager who delivered our drinks to the table.

At one point in the evening, the manager asked me how old I was. I looked down at my Bloody Mary and purposely didn't answer. I was having a good time with Moish and didn't want to scare him away, so I turned my head away from the nosy manager and focused my gaze on the band playing on stage.

Moish was interesting to talk to, a great conversationalist, funny, and intelligent—but it was his smile that I fell in love with that night. He had two huge dimples, and I would soon learn that even in his high school yearbook he had been nicknamed "Smiley." Although he acted cheerful, outspoken, and adventurous, Moish confided to me that he had been awkwardly shy as a young boy. He spent most of his early years with his parents and sister, and had very few close friends. He didn't blossom until high school, as evidenced by the fact that he got so many girls to go out with him.

***

Moish and I were married in 1973, and shortly thereafter moved into a beautiful house in Flatbush, a neighborhood in Brooklyn. Every morning Moish and I ate breakfast together, after which he would ride into Manhattan by train. After amicably parting ways with his father, Moish began working for a large CPA firm called N. Tannenbaum and Company. He started out on the bottom rung of the ladder, but after a few years he performed so well that they hired him on as partner.

Our house in Flatbush was in the perfect location—close to the grocery store, close to the synagogue, close to everything we could possibly need. I grew to love our house and neighborhood, and not just because my first five children were born there.

Our first child, Zevi, was born in 1974. Moish and I were ecstatic—he loved babies as much as I did. When I told him on one of our first dates that I wanted twelve children, Moish didn't flinch. It wasn't for religious reasons that I wanted so many kids; I had simply always desired the loving chaos that comes from having a large family.

The following year I gave birth to Ruchi, our oldest daughter. Two years later, in 1977, our second daughter Malkie was born, meaning that all of a sudden Moish and I found ourselves the proud parents of three kids under three. Our days—and nights—were filled with sleepless nights, crying babies, dirty diapers, and temper tantrums, but neither Moish nor I would have had it any other way.

The Seventies began as an idyllic time for Moish and me. We were a fun-loving couple, young and happy and energetic, enjoying time with our kids and our family. Unfortunately, not long after Malkie blessed our lives, we were suddenly confronted with a real-life tragedy.

Moish's mother, who was in her fifties, developed cancer. We were very close to her, and her sickness devastated our entire family. Her cancer progressed quickly, and only two years after her diagnosis, my precious mother-in-law passed away.

While Moish and I were still grieving over her loss, I became pregnant with our fourth child. The moment the obstetrician confirmed that I was pregnant, I knew in my heart it would be a girl. I wanted to name her after Moish's mother, but I was aware that this decision was bound to invite some complications.

In the Jewish tradition, it is customary to name a child after somebody who has already passed on. Our dilemma was that my own mother, who was very much alive, shared a name with Moish's mother. I thought she might be uncomfortable having me name my daughter after somebody who was still alive. To my pleasant surprise, my mother took Moish and I aside and assured us that she didn't have a problem with it.

My grandmother, on the other hand, was not pleased with the idea.

I told Moish how much I wanted to name our daughter after his mother, and after tearfully discussing it for several nights, Moish and I arrived at a solution that we prayed my grandmother would be amenable to.

"If we give our daughter a second name and call her *both* names, would you be okay with that?" we asked her.

Thankfully, my grandmother liked that idea, so when my daughter was born we named her Nechama Miriam. *Nechama* is the Hebrew word for comfort. For the many years my grandmother was alive, we called my daughter by both names.

It turned out that Miriam was a huge comfort to Moish's father, who spent many happy hours cradling her in his arms. My father-in-law was a Holocaust survivor who had lost his wife and two children in Auschwitz. For several years his life was pure hell. After the war, he married a lovely woman— Moish's mother—who was ten years younger than he was.

Never in his most terrible dreams did he imagine that she would pass away before he did.

***

At the beginning of the new decade, I found myself physically and mentally exhausted. Moish and I had four lovely and energetic children, and we were still reeling from the death of his mother. We needed a break, so we spent the next four years enjoying our young family and enjoying each other. Moish worked hard at the office while I worked hard at home, raising our children.

In 1984, our son Pinky was born. We named him after my beloved older brother, who had died years earlier from a sudden aneurism, leaving behind five children and his wife pregnant with twins. Pinky was the oldest child in our family and I was the youngest, so he was naturally overprotective of me, serving as my main confidant during my teenage years. When Pinky died my heart broke, and I often thought of him when I swaddled my newborn son.

During that time, Moish was working extremely long hours at N. Tannenbaum and Company, especially during tax season, when he often didn't return home until ten o'clock. Moish had always been enthusiastic about everything relating to religion—he frequently studied the Torah, and faithfully attended synagogue. At home, our family devoutly observed the Sabbath. I loved Moish's religious passion, and did everything I could to support him.

To complement this passion, Moish loved the land of Israel, and for five years, he had confided in me his dream of selling our house in Flatbush and moving permanently to Israel.

Part of me was intrigued by the idea of moving to Israel, while another part of me was hesitant. After all, I was comfortable living in Flatbush. I loved our house, which was always full of life, and the neighborhood we lived in. I loved my kids' schools, and had made numerous friends.

Each time Moish brought up the subject, I would hem and haw and make excuses for why it wasn't the right time to pick up and move. Something softened in me after Pinky was born, however, because I finally agreed to uproot my family, and in fact my whole life, and move 5,700 miles across the Atlantic Ocean. As I packed up our home, I began getting more and more excited about living and raising our kids in Israel.

In 1985, we sold our beloved house of more than ten years, and Moish humbly and happily gave up his partnership at N. Tannenbaum. He, along with his father, was extremely enthusiastic about this next chapter of his life.

Moish's father *loved* Israel, and was so happy we were moving there that he gave us a huge and unexpected gift: two years' rent on a nice apartment, paid in advance.

Our first year in Israel was an adventure, and I found myself happy, enthusiastic, and idealistic. There was so much to show our children, so much to experience. My kids loved exploring the country, trying exotic foods, and listening (and learning) to the new and fabulous language.

By the second year, much of the novelty of the country had worn off for me. There were times, especially when Moish was at work and I was in charge of the kids, when I began to question our decision to move. I found myself daydreaming more and more about my friends and house back in Flatbush.

One of the hardest things about living in Israel was adjusting to Moish's work schedule. Despite my father-in-law's generous gift, and despite the lower cost of living, we still had five children to feed. In order to make enough money, Moish traveled back to New York for nine weeks every tax season, which ran from the beginning of February through the middle of April. He worked eighteen-hour days during this time and made enough money to support our family in Israel for a year, especially considering that we lived modestly and that our rent had been taken care of. Still, when Moish was overseas I was, for all intents and purposes, a single parent in a foreign country. My father-in-law spent time with us, as his own apartment was only a few blocks away from ours, but it wasn't the same. I needed Moish to be a father to his kids. I needed Moish to be my husband.

By the third year, my unsettled feelings had morphed into a downright depression. I couldn't cope with my emotions living in Israel. Things were just too different. I missed my friends in New York, I missed my extended family, and I missed my house.

In truth, I missed *everything*.

To top it off, during Moish's last time away, I was pregnant with our sixth child, and was having difficulty hiding my feelings from my kids, who weren't even teenagers yet. When Moish returned to Israel, they told him: "I don't think Mommy's in great shape; you should do something about it."

Moish was devastated, but he understood my feelings. He had grown very attached to Israel. He loved the pace of life, and he loved that he had more time to study Torah— thankfully, his top priority was my happiness, so he agreed we would all move back in one year. One morning I asked my oldest son Zevi, who was finishing eighth grade, what he thought about returning to New York in a year.

"It's going to be hard for me to move back after I start high school," he told me. "If we do move back, it would be better to return in a few weeks so that I can begin high school in America."

Zevi was right, but once we officially decided to move back to New York, we found ourselves in a time crunch. We wanted to get settled in New York before school started in September. In a manic six-week period we sold our apartment in Israel and, with the help of my brother-in-law, a lawyer, purchased my friend's house in Brooklyn. I had seen the house years before, so I had a fair idea what it looked like. That was a stressful time for all of us—but for me it was a positive kind of stress, because I knew it would end with us living close to our extended families.

To add to the "good stress" in our lives, just before leaving Israel I gave birth to Perry. We named Perry after my grandmother, an act that caused me lots of reflection, especially living in Israel. A majority of my friends and neighbors there had lost their grandparents in the concentration camps in World War II. I was one of the rare and lucky ones who actually *knew* my maternal grandparents.

Moish and I only lived in Israel for three years, but moving back to New York was a huge adjustment, especially for our children. Pinky, for instance, was only four years old, so he knew *nothing* about America. In Israel we lived in a neighborhood where the majority of people observed the Sabbath and there was minimal traffic on Saturdays. Now he was living in the middle of Brooklyn, with its diversity and its constant honking of horns and round-the-clock noise. Everywhere Pinky looked he was confronted by some new and shocking experience.

In Israel there was a fancy hotel called The Plaza. It served meat, which was very expensive. Moish and I took Pinky there one afternoon for a treat; he loved it so much that he devoured an entire steak. When we returned to New York, I took Pinky to the King's Plaza shopping mall in Brooklyn, not far from our house. We looked in some stores and shared some cookies, but when we headed back to the car Pinky started crying. When I asked him what was wrong, he looked at me with his big, watery eyes and said, "Where's my steak?" It broke my heart.

Pinky wasn't the only one of my children who had trouble adjusting to the States. Even though I had the older kids tutored

11

in English while we were in Israel, I was realistic enough to know that tutoring alone wouldn't get them up to par. To a child of nine or ten, being away from America even for three years was apt to make things very difficult.

Shortly after we returned, Malkie had an English test at school. She studied hard for it, and knew the material backwards and forwards, but that afternoon when she came home from school she told me guiltily that she hadn't gotten a single question correct.

"That's not possible," I insisted. "I asked you every question and you answered them all correctly."

"I don't read script," Malkie cried. She had been too embarrassed to ask her teacher for help. Things like that were huge adjustments, both for me and my kids.

Moish, on the other hand, seemed to get back in the swing of things more quickly than the rest of us (perhaps since he had spent two months in New York every tax season). Which was not to say that everything went smoothly for him. Before our travels to Israel he had been an established partner in a large CPA firm, whereas now he was working for himself.

The four-story house we had bought was large enough for our expanding family, but it was also in desperate need of repairs. The important thing to us was that it was affordable, and Moish and I knew that over time, we could fix it up to our liking.

Moish and I slowly settled into our new home and neighborhood. Our house was constantly full of kids, especially on Friday nights, because our kids' friends would come over. Our house was known as the "cool house," full of unhealthy snacks and goodies, and many kids in the neighborhood knew it. It was filled with love and fun laughter and noise, and Moish and I were blessed to enjoy that house for more than twenty-five years.

***

Moish often learned Gemara (the second part of the Talmud) well into the night; his thirst to learn was impressive, yet before our trip to Israel Moish wouldn't have had the confidence to *teach* about the Talmud.

Back in New York, Moish frequently worried about not making enough money to support our growing family (I was pregnant with our seventh child, Sruly, at the time), so one day he sought out the wisdom of a well-respected rabbi, Rabbi Pam, whom he had known and felt close to for many years. When Moish asked him how to improve his livelihood, Rabbi Pam answered cryptically:

"I think you should teach the class on the Talmud."

"I don't think you heard my question," Moish responded, but when he repeated himself two more times, Rabbi Pam gave the same answer: "I think you should teach the class on the Talmud."

The class he was referring to—the *daf yomi*—is significant to the Jewish community because learners all around the world study the same single page of the Talmud on the same day. The entire study takes more than seven years to complete, and at the end of the study people worldwide celebrate the hard work they've put in—this celebration is called the *Siyum HaShas*.

The *daf yomi* is intense, complicated learning, and once we returned from Israel, Moish dedicated himself to creating time each day to study the Talmud. Moish was friends with a handful of men who were equally interested in the Talmud, so he started teaching the *daf yomi* class at 5:30 every morning at our dining room table. These men all had jobs, so it was the only time they could attend. Moish didn't mind—he woke up every morning at 3:00 to prepare diligently for that day's class.

As hard as he prepared for each day's lesson, however, Moish was self-conscious about teaching the class.

"I'm getting up early because I want to be well-prepared," he confided in me, "but why are these other people coming?"

Moish taught his class seven days a week until I asked him to take one day off. Moish graciously agreed to take off Saturday, the Sabbath. Saturday became my day… to read, to relax, to pray, and to spend time with Moish and my children.

***

Sruly was born in 1989, two years after Perry. The following year, at the dawn of the new decade, our final child Yitzy was born. Moish and I now headed up a family of ten, and our house was a constant den of love and laughter and chaos, but even eight children didn't tell the entire story of how busy and loud our house was.

Moish and I never formally adopted any children or brought in any official foster children, but throughout the years we housed several *unofficial* foster children. Some stayed for weeks, some stayed for months, and one stayed for nearly two years. I was passionate about taking in any child who needed a loving home, and Moish appreciated this quality about me. Although there was no question the primary responsibility for these extra kids lay with me (Moish was busy preparing for and teaching the *daf yomi* class), I was grateful that Moish allowed me to indulge my habit of bringing kids into our home, even if he wasn't as involved in their lives as I was.

Once Yitzy started elementary school, I began working part-time as a nurse at HASC, the Hebrew Academy for Special Children, in Brooklyn. There I had the privilege of spending my day with children with special needs—everything from genetic disabilities, to cerebral palsy, to autism. HASC housed between fifty and eighty children—aged five to twenty-one—at any given time, half of whom went home at the end of the day, and half of whom lived in group homes.

I loved going into work every day, and felt a connection with the kids and the other people who worked there. Many of my co-workers didn't work at HASC only for the money, but because they had huge hearts and were warm and loving people. We would celebrate many occasions with cupcakes, donuts, or other treats.

The kids provided me with a special perspective on life no matter how rotten a mood I was in, or how much traffic there had been on the drive to work, or how annoyed I might have gotten at Moish, as spouses sometimes do. The kids at HASC did things that warmed my heart and made it so I couldn't imagine working anywhere else. There was one boy without hands who gleefully played with toys using his elbows. There was another young girl with a terminal illness who laughed every time she heard her teacher's voice. These kids had a profound impact on my life, and I felt a deep empathy with their parents. I must admit, though, that I never felt the parents' *pain* with such magnitude until I started taking care of Moish.

***

For the first thirty years of our marriage, Moish and I embraced the chaos of raising eight children, of Moish waking up early in the morning to prepare for his *daf yomi* class, and of all the normal ups and downs couples have. For the first thirty years of our marriage, there was no sign of the dark times that Moish and I would eventually go through… except for one terrible incident 30,000 feet in the air, ten years before Moish got sick. What happened aboard that airplane was about as dark as it gets.

In the late Nineties, when my daughter Malkie married and relocated to Chicago, Moish and I decided to visit her. We spent a pleasant few days with Malkie and Abe, eating out at fabulous restaurants, laughing about the good times when

15

Malkie was growing up. Moish and I crammed a lot into two or three days, and we told Malkie and Abe we would visit again soon. We boarded our return flight to New York—which should have been an easy two-hour jaunt, enough to eat a bag of chips and drink a soda—knowing we'd be back home by dinnertime.

I leaned back to read a magazine, every so often marveling at the clouds outside our window. Moish was quiet, but his silence didn't strike me as anything out of the ordinary.

Once we had reached cruising altitude, Moish finally spoke.

"I'm not feeling so good," he told me. "I'm feeling a little bit nauseated."

I looked over at Moish, who did look peaked, but I assumed he was being dramatic, so I didn't think much about it.

Without warning, Moish's head slumped over, and his pillow and book fell to the floor. He was pale and appeared to be totally unconscious. I immediately went into shock. My body tingled and my heart pounded hard in my chest as I reached over and felt for Moish's pulse.

I couldn't find his pulse.

My first instinct was to pray and to find out if there was a doctor on the plane. I opened my mouth to ask the oblivious people in the surrounding seats, but I was so panicked that I could barely whisper, much less speak.

"Is anybody here a doctor?" I whispered, in an inexplicably calm and quiet voice. My body language clearly wasn't communicating the urgency that I felt.

"I need a doctor," I said, more loudly this time.

Praise *Hashem*, there was a doctor on board, and he gently pulled Moish out of his seat and lowered him into the middle of the aisle. When he took Moish's blood pressure, I could see the worry in his eyes.

"It's one hundred," the doctor said.

"One hundred over what?" I said.

"One hundred over nothing," he said.

My entire body tensed in panic—I felt like the whole world was slowing down. I couldn't believe that only two hours ago Moish was hugging his daughter goodbye at the airport coffee shop, and now he was lying in the middle of an airplane aisle, possibly dying.

I began praying, trying to make a deal that would keep my husband from becoming the lead story on that evening's national news.

Moish has started giving his class… and it's really important to him. I know it's only three people around a table right now, but it's going to grow. It's going to be a really important class. I promise you I'll never bother him about it. I won't interrupt him. This class means a lot to people, and he'll make it grow. Please let Moish live.

The doctor looked up, stone-faced, and asked the stewardess if there was a defibrillator on the plane. She said there wasn't; that was back in the archaic days before every flight came equipped with a defibrillator. The doctor told the stewardess that they needed to land the plane immediately—he told her that Moish had no pulse and no blood pressure. She scurried away to the front of the plane to inform the pilots, then returned minutes later to tell us they were going to land the plane in Buffalo.

I heard their words, but I wasn't really listening. In my head I was still frantically pleading for *Hashem* to intervene.

Please don't let him die. Please don't let my Moish die.

I looked down at my husband, ignoring the horrified stares of the other passengers. Moish's eyes were closed, and he didn't appear to be moving. Every few seconds I grabbed his arm, but I still couldn't feel a pulse.

"Moish," I pleaded. "If you know I'm here, squeeze my hand."

I felt a very light squeeze.

I looked at the doctor hopefully.

"He's here," I said. "Moish squeezed my hand. He's okay."

The doctor continued to work on Moish while I continued to talk with *Hashem*—I was in mid-thought when Moish's eyes slowly fluttered open. He was pale and visibly weak, but somehow, he got his voice back. The whispers of the surprised passengers grew louder. After a few minutes, Moish allowed us to raise him to his feet. For the first time I looked at the other passengers, and wondered if they were upset at us because their plane was landing in Buffalo instead of at LaGuardia.

American Airlines was very professional about the whole ordeal, and they managed to whisk us away from the scene without intrusion or embarrassment. They had an ambulance waiting for us on the tarmac in Buffalo, and it sped us off to the emergency room.

In the ambulance, for one of the rare times in my life, I was speechless. I didn't know if Moish's heart had given out, whether he had suffered a stroke, or whether he'd had some sort of brain seizure. Moish was as unsure about what had happened as I was.

The doctors at the hospital ran a full battery of worrisome tests, but ultimately insisted that everything looked okay. They released Moish after securing our promise that we would follow up with our physician as soon as we got back to Brooklyn.

When I called my kids to tell them what had happened—and that their father was going to be okay—my son-in-law Dovi surprised me by telling me that he had heard about the plane on the news, and that he had known instinctively that the distressed passenger was Moish. He didn't sound surprised at all.

Moish and I took a taxi ride from the emergency room back to the airport. I kept hugging him in the back of that cab, saying how ecstatic I was that he was alive. We were so preoccupied with our celebration that we almost missed our next flight, and had to run like lunatics through the airport to make it.

Once we were safely back on the second plane—which should have been more terrifying than it was—Moish told me he had been fully aware of everything that was happening. He told me he had worried that the doctor was going to crack his ribs with the defibrillator. I told him that a few cracked ribs would have been a small price to pay for not dying on the airplane.

We arrived home to our answering machine full of panicked messages from our kids; they had assumed we were going to call them again, and were imagining the worst, whereas I thought that one call was enough for the time being.

Moish woke up the next morning feeling tired but otherwise normal, but that didn't stop me from making appointments with a hundred different doctors. After shuttling Moish from doctor to doctor and having dozens of tests performed, the only thing that raised an eyebrow was an abnormal brain pattern.

Our neurologist in Brooklyn told us that Moish had a seizure disorder. He dutifully prescribed some anti-seizure medication and, much to Moish's horror, told Moish he couldn't drive.

Moish loved to drive, and was more upset about the driving ban than he was about having to take some new medication, even though that medication made him extremely sick. The medication made Moish so miserable that eventually he announced to me that he wanted to get on with his life, so he stopped taking it. I was worried but supportive of his decision, and for the next eight years, Moish didn't have a single seizure.

We were surprised years later to find out that he never had a seizure disorder.

Moish was thrilled to get back behind the wheel, but he and I were equally hesitant to get back on an airplane. For my part, I was hysterical even on the ground. Several times a week I would shake Moish awake in the middle of the night, checking his breathing, thinking he was dying; inevitably, I would be reminded about how suddenly my brother Pinky had died at the young age of thirty.

I was a complete wreck, even though Moish believed that everything was fine. He even stubbornly refused to take part in some of the doctors' tests, such as one where they wanted to hang him upside down for twenty minutes. Moish was more adaptable than I was, more willing to embrace change, and over time I took a clue from Moish's optimism and tried not to think about his condition—it took about a year until I was able to put it out of my head.

Of course, sometimes late at night I would still think about our ordeal on the airplane, and would get frustrated because I had no clue what had happened, and had no clue *why* it had happened. All I really knew was that I was overjoyed that it never happened again.

CHAPTER 2

When people think about dementia, most of them think only about the loss of memory—but the disease is so much more sinister than that. Those who have not witnessed dementia first hand don't understand the serious *psychiatric* components of the disease—anxiety, fear, and paranoia. They don't understand how all of the victim's emotions became exaggerated, the good and the bad.

Sadly, in the years following the plane incident, I experienced *all* of these with Moish. And others did, too.

My mother—who had macular degeneration and who spent many weekends with us—struck a nerve one night after dinner when she watched Moish clearing away the dishes. She said to me with a smirk, "Since when is your husband clearing off the table? Since when is Moish helping so much?"

Despite my annoyance with her comment, I had to admit my mother was right—Moish seemed to be compensating for something. He had always been a kind, helpful man, but he had recently become even kinder. For instance, now when Moish saw somebody on the street he wanted to help them, even if it was a complete stranger.

This dramatic change in Moish's behavior wasn't contained to him; it affected me as well.

At Sruly's bar mitzvah in 2003, Moish was shuffling around, demonstrably irritated about everything… even about trivial things like the cake. Our son's bar mitzvah should have been one of the greatest days of Moish's life, but he wasn't enjoying the moment like he normally would have. His attitude was depressingly negative, and as a result I felt like *I* was going to blow a gasket. In 2003, I was 49 years old and Moish was 54.

In desperation, I asked my sister-in-law for a sedative.

"Give me anything," I begged. "I don't care what it is. I can't lose my temper today."

I knew that if I got angry with Moish, we'd end up having a huge, blow-up fight… and that would be the end of the happy bar mitzvah. So I took my sister-in-law's sedative, even though I'd never taken one in my life.

Later that day, Ruchi's father-in-law pulled her aside and told her I looked drugged.

"Oh, she definitely is," Ruchi laughed.

Her father-in-law laughed, too; fortunately, Ruchi's in-laws were the types who could handle it.

***

Then there was Moish's unfounded, completely exaggerated paranoia, the best example of which occurred when my daughter Perry, then about sixteen years old, was standing on our front porch, waiting to be picked up by a friend. In our neighborhood, we always told our kids that at night it was safer to have a second person with you.

On this particular evening, Perry's friend called to her from the corner, and she ran down and got in their car.

Moish went absolutely nuts.

"How could Perry do that?" he screamed.

"What did she do?" I asked.

"Perry knows she can't go anywhere alone!" Moish said. He was practically shaking he was so upset.

Moish was being completely irrational, and seemed unaware of the actual situation—that Perry's friend was on the corner, watching every step she took. Perry was safe, but Moish was acting like a band of marauders was breathing down her neck.

In addition to this near-constant paranoia, Moish tended to repeat his stories, although the details often got mixed up. My natural instinct was to correct him, but I wasn't willing to hurt him like that. As long as his story wasn't inappropriate or horrible, I never corrected him, even if what he was saying was off-the-charts ridiculous.

Needless to say, Moish's confusion negatively began to impact our social life. Soon I could count on a single hand the number of people I felt we could comfortably socialize with. I had confided in several people about Moish's condition, so I felt comfortable going over to their houses.

The truth was, I was exasperated by the changes I saw in Moish, and there were very few people outside of my family I wanted to share a meal with. They had to be people who were kind to Moish and who went out of their way to make him feel comfortable. Sadly, as time went on, fewer and fewer people seemed to fall into that category.

***

In 2005, Pinky began dating a beautiful woman named Miri. Over the course of time, like all couples do, Pinky described the members of his family to her. We had the pleasure of meeting Miri shortly before their engagement. When she finally met us, she pulled Pinky aside and told him, to his surprise: "Everybody here is exactly like you described them… except for your father."

Pinky didn't live at home anymore, so he didn't see it as clearly, but the man Pinky had grown up with was *not* the same man Miri met. I began noticing changes in Moish—some subtle, some not so subtle—as far back as 2003, five years before his official diagnosis. Most of those changes were behavioral—for instance, he was very tense. Moish also wasn't as funny as he had been years before or, sadly, as adorable. Our kids didn't always see this for what it was.

On numerous occasions I was irritated with Moish because I thought he was acting strange on purpose. I shudder to think how many times I said things that, in retrospect, were hurtful. When I told Moish I thought he was acting weird, he was very defensive. At the time, I didn't know whether those incidents were serious or not—although that horrible episode on the plane was *always* in the back of my mind.

I wasn't content to let Moish's behavior go unchecked, so aside from seeing medical professionals, I asked people to give blessings for Moish. Although I feverishly researched Moish's symptoms online every night, I wasn't averse to asking *Hashem* for help as well—I would take whatever help I could get. One very wise rabbi advised me that if I were truly praying for a miracle for Moish, I *shouldn't* make a public announcement about it. I dutifully kept my mouth shut for about a year. I am wired to talk to everybody I meet, so it went against my nature to stay quiet about something as important as my husband's health, and I was extremely nervous.

Of all the changes I saw in Moish, the most noticeable was how nervous he was. This brought about an internal conflict with how I saw my family versus how others saw us. I considered my family to be emotional and passionate and loud—but not nervous. I was taken aback when one of my sons-in-law good-naturedly began calling us "the nervous

Friedmans." After some soul-searching, I had to admit to myself that Moish and I both *were* nervous and high-strung; but once Moish got sick, *his* nervousness careened out of control.

At first, I didn't attribute this to sickness. I attributed it to the fact that Moish was getting up at 3:00 in the morning to teach his *daf yomi* class and only slept three or four hours a night—unhealthy by any measure. I thought that perhaps lack of sleep might be the culprit. I thought that perhaps Moish was having a nervous breakdown, but I didn't think at the beginning that it might be a neurodegenerative disease.

Some of the incidents were subtle—Moish worrying about insignificant things—while others were embarrassing and worrisome. One of these latter incidents occurred at the wedding of my nephew Phil. Moish drank a single glass of wine, but was acting as though he had ten.

I kept an eye on Moish as I greeted friends and family and then watched, horrified, as he tried to take a rose out from one of the centerpieces. He intended to do some sort of flamenco dance with the rose in his mouth, which admittedly would have been cute and charming, but when he reached for the rose, he destroyed the entire centerpiece. That was entirely against Moish's nature and, watching dumbstruck as he attempted to clean up the mess, I knew that the only explanation was that he was drunk.

I felt like I was the only one at the wedding who *wasn't* laughing—everybody else seemed to find Moish's behavior funny. Objectively, I suppose, Moish *was* being funny, but he wasn't acting like my husband. Moish barely drank, and he certainly never got drunk to the point of creating a scene at a wedding.

When I confronted Moish about his behavior, he responded by getting angry with me.

"You never let me have any fun," Moish pouted. "I'm going home with Zevi."

I didn't know what to say; leaving a wedding early without me was very unlike him.

Before he left, I motioned Zevi over to me.

"It's not true, is it?" I whispered. "Dad didn't have just one glass of wine?"

Zevi looked at the floor, as if he were debating how to answer.

"He only had one," Zevi said.

"Something's not right," I told him. Zevi gave me a hug that told me that he knew, as I did, that Moish was not acting like himself.

When I told Zevi that something wasn't right with his father, I meant it. Nothing about the incident made sense to me, and I bawled the entire drive home.

It wasn't until years later that it occurred to me that if something is wrong with your brain, then even *one glass* of alcohol can cause things to go badly.

***

Shortly after the incident at Phil's wedding, Moish began acting out his dreams in the middle of the night. He did this often—some nights I would lie awake for hours watching him.

Late one night, Moish's hand began to jerk, almost as if he were having a seizure. I intertwined our fingers, wondering if that would help.

It didn't.

Instead, Moish's foot began to jerk, and his face looked as unhappy as I'd ever seen it.

When he yelled, I flinched and woke him up.

"Are you dreaming?" I asked him.

Moish nodded that he was.

"Do you remember your dream?" I asked.

"Yes," Moish said. "Sammy and I were being chased by somebody. We tried to hide near a rock so he couldn't catch us."

As Moish slowly calmed down, I realized he had been acting out his dreams for quite a while. Frequently he was frightened in his dreams, which I couldn't relate to, as I generally dreamed about things that were frustrating, like not being able to get to work on time.

When Moish screamed or cried out in his sleep, I would gently wake him up and try to calm him down. When he talked in his sleep, his voice was loud and clear. This was sometimes accompanied by jerky arm, leg, and body movements. Other times Moish's fear was replaced by anger, and he would thrash around and yell in his sleep.

One common theme for Moish was that he dreamed about things that had happened to him the day before. One time, at 4:30 in the morning, Moish began screaming about trial balances.

"Let me finish my sentence!" he yelled.

The day before, I had given our taxes to our accountant. I wanted to fax her a letter that we had received regarding our tax information; it was completely insignificant, but Moish got upset when he saw it.

"Do you realize you're paying for her time?" he asked me. "Why don't you show it to me first—maybe I can do it."

I told Moish that we had already talked about how he couldn't do the return, and that the letter was just one unimportant piece of paper, but he got furious with me. I felt sad for him—as well as for myself.

Another night, Moish dreamed he was at a wedding—he was singing the tunes and having conversations with people. The previous night Moish and I had attended a wedding, so obviously it was on his mind.

Sometimes when Moish acted out his dreams I was tempted to video him, but I decided that would be degrading. His actions were impossible to describe, however, and I had a need to share Moish's strange behavior with someone. In the end, I couldn't go through with it. I had too much respect for what Moish was going through to capture it on video.

***

Having eight children, our house at times tended more toward *disorder* than order. Keeping things neat and tidy is hard enough with no kids, but when your house is "the place to be" for the neighborhood kids, trying to keep things organized is beyond difficult, especially during the holidays.

This lack of organization didn't bother me until Moish began getting confused. This confusion was undoubtedly exacerbated by the lack of structure in our household. One day, for instance, Moish went to synagogue wearing a jacket from one suit and pants from another. I explained to my kids that if they left their jackets laying around, Moish would assume they were his and wear them out in public.

When Moish and I were alone, I worked extremely hard to keep things orderly so he wouldn't get confused or agitated, but I learned the hard way that it was nearly impossible with a house full of people.

In the same vein, I also decided to fix some of the broken things around the house, even though we were woefully low on money. In desperation, I dipped into our 401(k); part of me knew that wasn't a smart thing to do, because I would have to pay a penalty for taking an early withdrawal, but the broken things around my house were getting on my nerves.

I wasn't doing any of this to beautify our home—I was afraid *not* to fix anything related to plumbing or electricity. In the back of my head, I imagined one day having to sell our home, and I knew it needed to be in the best condition possible. I didn't have the money and I was tired of asking people for money, so I took it out of our IRA, despite the penalties. I fervently believed it was worth paying a small penalty to have some peace of mind.

***

Starting in 2006, Moish and I spent much of our time going to different neurologists, which was more frustrating than I had anticipated. On our very first visit, the neurologist said that Moish was fine, and advised us to leave things alone and let nature take its course. On our second visit to the neurologist, I insisted that Moish was *far* from being fine. The neurologist told me the only diagnosis he was willing to give was mild cognitive impairment, which might or might not eventually lead to dementia.

I became upset because I felt the neurologist wasn't taking me seriously. I was a trained nurse who was with Moish all the time, and I was extremely worried.

Frustrated, I went to visit Moish's first cousin, Dr. Avi Leb, a physician with a heart of gold. He was willing to listen to everything I had to say. Avi told me that we first needed to rule out any sort of physical cause of Moish's symptoms. I made a comprehensive list, and was ultimately able to rule out most physical factors.

After that, I knew for certain I needed to find another neurologist who would listen closely to what I was saying. What I wasn't aware of at the time was that not all neurologists are created equal, and that each neurologist has his or her own specialty, whether that be seizures, or memory disorders, or multiple sclerosis.

While making a list of Moish's symptoms, one thing that occurred to me was that when Moish fell asleep—even at the table or in his living room chair—his head would slump over, and no matter how hard I tried, I couldn't wake him up.

Maybe he had sleep apnea, I thought. I made an appointment with someone who specialized in sleep disorders. I wasn't surprised one bit when he diagnosed Moish with sleep apnea and prescribed one of those horrible CPAP machines to help Moish breathe. Moish was willing to try the machine and I was hopeful, but after several weeks of wearing it, there was no change either in Moish's sleep patterns or his general behavior. Disappointed that the CPAP machine wasn't the solution to our problem, we moved on to the next neurologist, who specialized in seizures.

This neurologist diagnosed Moish with a seizure disorder, which thrilled me because if it was a seizure disorder, they could help Moish with medication. I told my kids what the neurologist said, and they were as ecstatic as I was.

The only person who wasn't dancing for joy was Moish, who turned to me and asked, "Why are you so happy?"

"It's a good diagnosis," I told him. "It's treatable."

"How do you know the diagnosis is right?" Moish said.

Throughout our life, I thought that I was more of an optimist than Moish—regardless, I was surprised that he was questioning the diagnosis. Perhaps Moish didn't believe the doctor, or perhaps he was thinking back to the incident on the plane, when the seizure medication they prescribed made him so miserably sick.

***

When people hear that I'm a nurse, they often ask me to diagnose the new mole they have on their arm, or to feel their lymph nodes to see if they're swollen, or to ask about various symptoms. In Moish's case, having medical knowledge was a double-edged sword. While I was able to help Moish in certain situations, my mind also went haywire every time Moish exhibited a new symptom. A dozen different and often contradictory diagnoses swirled around constantly in my head.

The truth was, I didn't know what was wrong with Moish, but I did know with absolute certainty that *something* was wrong with him, and I became very, very worried.

In the spring of 2006, Moish and I took a trip to Israel in order to visit our parents' graves. Every few years, Moish and I traveled to Israel to pay respect to our parents and to my brother who were buried there, and to tour some of the historical religious sites.

On this trip, the historical religious sites didn't interest me in the least. I didn't want to take a tour; in fact, I didn't want to make any plans at all. For me, this trip was only about one thing—praying for Moish's health and my sanity. I wanted to pray at some of the holy places, and to ask for blessings from some of the holy rabbis.

That was an emotional visit for us, and in some dark part of my mind, I feared it might be our last trip together to Israel. It turned out to be a beautiful trip, peaceful, serene, and reflective. Moish and I spent our time being together and praying.

Even in his altered state, Moish knew that I was worried. I wasn't particularly adept at keeping my fears to myself, although I never intentionally spelled things out for Moish unless he asked. I could see on his face that he was worried too, although not anywhere near the level that I was.

One thing I worried about were skills that Moish used to be good at, such as following directions. I was born with a terrible sense of direction, while Moish had the uncanny ability of looking at a map and getting us anywhere.

It was very noticeable—and very scary—when his ability changed. Moish still *tried* to get us places, but he would tell me to make a left turn when I was positive I needed to turn right. I didn't fight him, even when I was one hundred percent certain he was wrong. I knew Moish would eventually figure out that I was correct, but I made a conscious decision not to *tell* Moish he was wrong, since he had no control over it.

The situation with directions got so bad that we went to see a handful of neurologists about it, but every one of them dismissed it; I'm convinced they were "fooled" by Moish's intelligence and poise, and by the fact that he could hold a beautiful conversation with them. He simply didn't come across as the kind of man who had a degenerative disease. When I insisted that something was seriously wrong with Moish, one neurologist looked at me curiously, as if *I* were the one losing my mind.

***

It's common when you have a sick spouse to question *why* it happened. Was it hereditary? Or was it simply *Hashem's* will that they be stricken with their affliction?

When we lived in Israel, Moish and I met a very interesting couple, Aurohom and Rochel Schwartzbaum, whom I found myself drawn to. They were both brilliant—he was a Fulbright Scholar—and had lived interesting lives. Unable to have children of their own in their first few years of their marriage, they adopted a young girl from China and wrote a book, *The Bamboo Cradle,* about their struggles converting their daughter to Judaism.

In Israel, I hired Rochel's daughter Devora to tutor my kids in English so they wouldn't fall behind if we ever moved back to New York. Devora and I were very close when she moved to Baltimore, Maryland, my hometown. We lost touch with each other somewhat, as people do, but reconnected when her father developed an inoperable brain tumor. Devora trusted me to give her advice, so she called me frequently throughout the difficult stages of her father's illness.

After her father passed (at which point Moish was already sick), Rochel confided in me that one thing that upset her children was that their father, a writer and a scholar, developed a brain tumor that affected his thinking process. One of her sons went so far as to ask a rabbi why his father's sickness specifically attacked his brain—the essence of who he was.

"Why would *Hashem* do that?" his son asked.

"Every person has something they want to accomplish in their life," the rabbi replied. "Sometimes you accomplish something in life that you're very good at... but then G-d gives you an opportunity to become stronger in other areas... maybe that's what it is."

I told Rachel that her story made me feel better because Moish was acting extremely emotional and sensitive, and that he was reaching out a lot to other people.

Moish's increased sensitivity was amazing for me to watch. He noticed things that I didn't notice. He felt badly that he had developed some severe limitations—both in and out of the house—which in turn made him more sensitive to others.

I told myself to accept this about Moish. He knew his sickness was a drain on me, and he tried hard to help me in areas where normally he would have been too busy. Even with simple chores like setting the table, Moish knew he was limited, and suddenly wanted to do all of those things.

CHAPTER 3

While Moish's sickness affected all of our children in different ways, his condition was particularly hard on Sruly, our second-youngest son, because their personalities were so similar. In both movement and thought, Sruly reminded me of Moish in a hundred different ways. Part of this was a religious fervor I couldn't relate to—Sruly's passion for learning the Talmud and for tackling the difficult religious questions of the day was eerily similar to what I had become used to in Moish.

Moish and Sruly loved nothing more than poring over Hebrew books. Sometimes the rest of us had no idea what they were talking about. This generally came to a boil on Friday nights, when Sruly and his father would get into animated, sometimes-heated religious discussions. They would block out the rest of the room, almost to the point of rudeness.

I used to wish that Moish and Sruly would involve all of us in their discussions… until they stopped. Over the course of a year or two, Sruly recognized how intellectually limited his father had become, and in many ways, he felt like he'd lost his partner. This transformation was painful to watch. Sruly didn't lose respect for his father, but it changed from a respect for Moish's knowledge into a respect for the fact that he was sick.

On Friday nights, Sruly and Moish weren't exclusive anymore. They weren't rude to the others, and I found myself missing that rudeness as soon as it was no longer there. Some of the others missed it too; Zevi confided to me that he felt as if he'd lost his best friend. That was already a lonely time for me in many ways because my five older children were all married and having beautiful Friday night meals with their own families.

***

Throughout our marriage, Moish was much more knowledgeable than me regarding the myriad laws of *Yom Tov* (the Jewish holidays), many of which are extremely intricate. I didn't need to memorize some of the more obscure laws by heart, because I knew that Moish would follow them to the letter. I relied on him to tell me what I needed to do—or not do—in any particular situation. Moish reminded me what foods I needed to buy and what preparations I needed to make before each holiday began.

Normally, in a case like ours, when a religious husband gets sick, the wife develops an attachment to a rabbi. In our specific situation, however, the rabbi I felt closest to had passed away (my husband's rabbi was Rav Pam, may he rest in peace). Rather than seeking out a new rabbi, I chose to rely on Zevi, who graciously and gracefully took over Moish's role in that regard.

In certain instances, I asked Zevi what laws I needed to follow, while in other instances I simply did what I thought was right. Out of emotional necessity, I often became *less* stringent during the holidays, which I found to be depressing once Moish became ill. We lived across the street from the synagogue, and watching the people there talking and socializing made me feel sad and lonely.

Sometimes people came by to say hello to Moish, although the number of visitors dwindled noticeably with each passing holiday. There were one or two blessed souls who stuck with him—I was so grateful for them. I also made a conscious effort *not* to be upset with those people who didn't visit anymore. I know that is the way of the world, and I'm quite sure that at times I was guilty of the same behavior.

***

After being diagnosed with a seizure disorder, I insisted that Moish take his prescribed medication for several months, even though I had to call the doctor a dozen times, explaining that the pills seemed to be *hurting* Moish, not helping him. The doctor repeatedly told me to give the medication time to work, but over time I wore him down, and he told me I could stop having Moish take any seizure medication at all.

Although I weaned Moish off the medicine *slowly*, it wasn't slow enough—and we found out the hard way that even if you don't have a seizure disorder, you can still have a seizure if you don't wean yourself from the medicine properly.

One morning, I received a call from Community Hospital in Brooklyn, informing me that my husband was in the emergency room after suffering a grand mal seizure on a city bus; it was classified as *status epilepticus*, an emergency situation in which the seizures don't stop. In a blind panic, I called my kids and told them to meet me at the hospital.

Working at HASC with special needs kids, I was no stranger to seizures; they were almost a daily occurrence there, and in most cases the normal treatment was to give the patient a drug called Ativan which, within minutes, stopped the seizure. Ativan was the same drug they were giving Moish through an IV in his arm, but for some reason, in Moish's case, it was literally making him psychotic.

I was living a nightmare. I was in a small local hospital I didn't feel comfortable in so, in desperation, I called Columbia and begged them to transfer Moish. He was already seeing the seizure specialist there. They told me in no uncertain terms that it would be completely unsafe to transfer Moish in the delicate condition he was in.

That's when things started to get interesting.

Zevi's mother-in-law, Malka Fass, graciously contacted someone to get in touch with Rav Chaim Kanievsky, a great rabbi living in Israel, to give Moish a blessing known as a *bracha*. Malka called to tell me that when her son-in-law explained Moish's situation to Rav Chaim, he gladly gave Moish a *bracha*.

Not five minutes later—which admittedly seemed like hours to me—I received a very surprising but welcome call from Columbia, telling me they were willing to admit Moish after all. I was overwhelmed with gratitude, and wondered whether I was experiencing divine guidance, a persuasive rabbi, or some sort of miracle. Either way, it was miraculous to me that Columbia would agree to accept a patient as unstable as Moish only five minutes after a rabbi 5,000 miles away gave us a blessing.

Grateful to Rav Chaim and to Malka, I stayed by Moish's side as he was transferred to the neurology ICU at Columbia. Moish was acting delirious, completely out of his mind, and neither we nor the doctors had any idea what was happening. All I knew for certain was that Moish was in terrible shape, and I didn't know if he was going to return home in the same condition as when he left. Like with so many things in life, it was the *not knowing* that was the hardest part.

From the very beginning, I had wanted to get Moish an appointment with a neurologist at Columbia who specialized in memory, but I couldn't get an appointment.

Here was my chance. Once Moish was settled in the ICU, I explained to the nurse how I'd been trying to make an appointment with their memory specialist, but that he was booked. I pleaded with her, asking if there was any way my husband could get in to see him.

"Definitely," the nurse said. "Just ask for a consultation with Doctor Horn."

I was shocked and delighted to secure an appointment with Dr. Horn. When we met he promised me that in a few weeks he would be able to give me some clarity on Moish's condition. I felt a sense of measured relief at this situation; after all, we had been running from doctor to doctor for two years, and nothing seemed to be getting better. I was happy we would be getting some sort of technical diagnosis that I could share with family and friends, many of whom *still* thought I was blowing Moish's condition out of proportion. They weren't seeing what I was seeing, and in many cases Moish appeared okay to them. But they weren't around him day in and day out, witnessing the episodes where Moish acted like a completely different person.

It was a tremendous relief talking to Dr. Horn, knowing that in a matter of time, we would finally know what we were dealing with.

***

I was impressed with Dr. Horn's medical knowledge and demeanor, but there was one thing about him that drove me absolutely crazy—I was hardly ever able to reach him on the telephone.

At first this was annoying, but eventually it became discouraging and depressing. He always had to be the one to reach out to me, meaning I had to carry my phone around twenty-four hours a day, even into the bathroom. If he called during one of the rare times I *didn't* have my phone, I'd have to wait an entire day or two to talk with him. On two occasions he called on the Sabbath or on holidays after I'd been trying to get hold of him for an entire week.

This upset me because the solution was easy—just give me a half-hour window once a week where I could call and touch base. This would have allowed me to save up my questions and ask them all at once. My inability to contact Dr. Horn, combined with the continuing lack of understanding from certain family and friends, was threatening to drive me mad.

The part that upset me the most about Dr. Horn's refusal to let me call him was that he understood me perfectly when I talked about Moish. He simply couldn't comprehend how traumatic it was for me not to be able to reach him in a timely manner; I could only call and leave a message and wait to hear back.

As provoked as I so often was, I wasn't quite ready to switch doctors, and I even rationalized the situation by telling myself that if I were spending much of *my* time working with hysterical, irrational caretakers, I might not give out my phone number either.

As a result of this lack of communication, and bolstered by my own training, I began researching and making medical decisions for Moish on my own. After getting frustrated with Dr. Horn and others, I made the conscious decision not to visit doctors anymore unless it was absolutely necessary.

There was only one roadblock to this—we were on Medicaid, which constantly required that we reveal when we last saw the doctor. To combat this, sometimes I bent the truth—for instance, sending a *picture* of Moish rather than seeing a doctor in person. If Moish had an infection on his leg, I could simply send a picture to the doctor so I didn't have to cart Moish down to the hospital.

In the back of my mind, I knew that if things ever got so serious I couldn't handle them, I could call an ambulance.

Where we lived in Brooklyn, however, it was usually easier to walk a few blocks to the hospital than to wait for an ambulance.

***

Moish's sickness often manifested itself with a terrible stabbing pain in his abdomen, usually on Friday night during the Sabbath. There was obviously some trigger about Friday nights—perhaps Moish was concerned that he wasn't functioning as the respectable person he used to be at synagogue, where people were impressed by his *daf yomi* class and considered him to be a knowledgeable, friendly man. The synagogue had long been the center of Moish's social network, so perhaps it was frightening to him because he wasn't the same person he had been in the past.

Physically, Moish's attacks looked like he had appendicitis—his face would go pale, and he would bend over and scream in pain. The first time it happened at 2:00 in the morning; I was woken out of a dead sleep to the sound of Moish's terrified screams. My first thought was that Moish was having a heart attack. I immediately gave him some medication and tried to calm him down. I tried to tell him the pain would go away, although I'm not sure either of us believed that at the moment.

I called Dr. Horn's service and said it was an emergency. I received a call-back shortly thereafter and asked if I should call an ambulance.

Doctor Horn began talking to me very slowly, very calmly—which did nothing to settle my own hysteria. I just thought, *Why are you so calm?*

"Can you hear Moish in the background?" I asked.

"I hear him," Dr. Horn assured me. "There's something we call a panic attack."

I couldn't believe it—my husband was doubled over in pain, white as a ghost, and my neurologist was diagnosing it as a simple panic attack.

"That's what this is?" I said incredulously. "How do you know? Maybe he's having… I don't know… something."

"This is what you're going to do," Dr. Horn replied, still infuriatingly calm. He gave me step-by-step instructions and told me everything was going to be okay. In a huff, I did everything he instructed me to do—and just like that, Moish's pain disappeared as quickly as it had come.

The next time Moish woke up doubled in pain—again, on a Friday night—I kept my emotions in check. I was still worried on the inside, but not nearly as much as the first time. I was able to deal with it on my own.

Over the next several months, Moish seemed to have an attack every few weeks. Sometimes I called Zevi to help me because, despite Dr. Horn's diagnosis, it was frightening to watch my husband in so much pain. Zevi always ran over, huffing and puffing, although by the time he arrived, Moish had usually calmed down and fallen back asleep.

A year or two after these attacks began, Moish needed to have his gallbladder removed, and I suspected that the two things were connected. I'll never know for sure, but undoubtedly there were several instances in which Moish was sick but simply couldn't explain his symptoms to me.

***

The initial diagnosis given to Moish was Early-onset Alzheimer's, which allowed me to form a plan of attack. I began reading every book and magazine article I could find on the subject. Researching Moish's sickness had a calming effect on me—a feeling that was bolstered by attending an amazing but sobering Alzheimer's conference in April of 2008. From the moment I set foot into the conference room, I felt that my feelings were being validated. After so much doubt and dismissal from the people in my life, I was finally around people who understood the pain and suffering Moish and I were feeling. I met people who had lost their spouses in their thirties and forties; I hadn't realized that people that young could get so sick. I found myself in tears during most of the conference, especially during the speeches.

My favorite speaker was a good-looking, highly educated bear of a man named Richard Taylor, who gave a touching speech about his own experiences and struggles with Early-onset Alzheimer's. I thanked him afterwards for his insights and powerful speech, and after I returned from the conference I continued to read his enlightening writings on the subject.

***

Several weeks later, I was finally beginning to wrap my head around Moish's diagnosis—but then experienced a gut-wrenching moment of frustration when Dr. Horn walked into the exam room, typing the results from Moish's spinal tap onto his computer.

"Oh, oh, oh," he said, with a furrowed brown; he was looking intently at his computer, not at Moish or me.

I looked at him, expectantly, and in that calm voice he had, Dr. Horn said: "You know, I think that Moish has Lewy Body Dementia."

Lewy Body Dementia?

I had never heard of such a thing, and I was a nurse.

"What is that?" I asked.

Dr. Horn explained that Lewy Body Dementia was the second most common degenerative disease behind Alzheimer's, even though most people had never heard of it.

When I got home I cried about the entire situation. I cried that our doctor was so casual when he announced this new diagnosis. I cried because he was completely oblivious to how much effort I had put in the last few weeks thinking Moish had something else.

I got over my shock, of course. I didn't have a choice. Moish had what he had, and my biggest dilemma became whether to tell people that Moish had Lewy Body Dementia, or just to tell them he had simple dementia.

Once I had cried all my tears, I appreciated the fact that I could finally give a name to Moish's illness. I could research it all day and all night. I could explain the diagnosis to my friends and family.

The real question, though, was whether I could *accept* the diagnosis.

CHAPTER 4

Despite being sick, Moish was somehow able to find humor in his situation, which made me wonder if he truly understood how terribly sick he was. I do know that at the beginning, he didn't comprehend how confused he was, and didn't realize how often he said strange and nonsensical things.

I rationalized this behavior by telling myself that if Moish indeed did have a brain disease, maybe he simply couldn't comprehend it. Would he be in such a good mood if he understood what was going on?

The bottom line was, Moish took his sickness better than anybody I ever met. I don't know why, and I don't know how, although I do know that his attitude was greatly helped by his faith.

"If this is what G-d wants for me, that's okay," he told me. "G-d is giving me the opportunity to fix anything I may have done wrong."

I couldn't believe that Moish was able to be so optimistic. He and I weren't on the same level at that point—I was struggling to accept my new position as caretaker, even though I knew that *Hashem* was doing everything for the best.

It was difficult for me to accept such a frightening prognosis, but I promised myself that I would try not to get upset at those people who loved us but didn't understand what we were going through. I promised myself I would try to accept that my financial stability—or, more precisely, my lack of it—was in G-d's hands. And I promised myself that even though I felt broken and hopeless every single day, I would try my hardest to act upbeat—for my coworkers, for my friends, and for my family.

Even though I didn't consider myself the most religious person in the world, I must have said ten thousand prayers along the way, although I didn't believe my prayers were going to help Moish become the first person to be cured from dementia. Of course, somebody, somewhere, *will* be that person, but I didn't think it would be us. Sometimes I laughed when somebody wished Moish a speedy recovery. Why were they saying that—didn't they know there was no cure? On the other hand, what else should they say?

I didn't believe that a miracle was going to occur, or that Moish was somehow going to get better. I prayed, of course, as did many others, but what *I* was praying for was that Moish would maintain his dignity, and that he wouldn't suffer. As long as Moish wasn't in physical pain, I was okay—I just didn't believe that anything past that was realistic.

***

A thousand things went through my mind when Dr. Horn gave us his startling diagnosis—the chief among them being how important it was to get rid of Moish's CPA practice. It had become our family's albatross, but it wasn't only about the money. Moish had passionately and skillfully built up his practice, step by step, over twenty years. He had developed and cultivated a beautiful reputation as a pleasant, conscientious, and trustworthy accountant, and I didn't want that reputation to go down the drain. I didn't want Moish to suffer any sort of public humiliation.

In short, I didn't want things to go to hell… although I had a feeling that I might be too late.

During that time, Moish was taking the bus to work every day. He would stay at the office for three or four hours, then ride the bus back home. I was nervous about this, always picturing the worst, so I asked his sister Perele if she would go into work with Moish to see how things were going.

To put it simply, things were *not* going well.

Moish was going into the office every day, but he wasn't getting anything productive done. To make matters worse, his mere presence in the office seemed to be causing problems for the other employees who, unfortunately, didn't know how to reveal to me how out of control things had gotten.

When Perele described the reality of the situation, I couldn't handle the news. On a practical level I needed to be aware of the things Moish was screwing up at the office, but on another level, my mind wasn't ready to hear it.

Finally, I visited the office myself and discovered that the situation was worse than I imagined—and I had imagined a complete disaster.

Moish couldn't accomplish even the simplest tasks. He couldn't log into his computer. He couldn't make copies or find simple documents. Sometimes he couldn't even remember what day or week or month it was.

Then there were the employees; all were dedicated and talented accountants, but they didn't necessarily understand how difficult this entire situation was. One young man was curious why Moish was asking him how to do certain things when it was Moish himself who had taught him. This man did not comprehend that Moish had *no memory* of teaching him.

On the few occasions that I was brave enough to venture into the office, I overheard the employees talking about Moish—and about me. On some level I understood what they were discussing, but I wished they would confront me directly. Perhaps they were waiting for me to confront them.

The last time I visited the office, I realized that Moish had to leave before he completely lost his dignity. It was painful to watch people doing mundane activities, wishing beyond hope that Moish was able to do the same.

I took Moish aside and told him it was time to bite the bullet and reach out to his clients. They had a right to know how bad things had gotten. It was time, I told him bluntly, to sell the practice, and I was startled but relieved when Moish agreed with me.

"I *want* to sell my practice," Moish insisted, "but if I start telling people I'm sick, this is going to get really bad. All my clients are going to leave, and then I'm not going to have anything left to sell. We have to wait until we find a buyer."

I knew Moish was right, but that didn't do anything to alleviate the constant stress I felt regarding our finances. After all, we had weddings to pay for and kids who needed health insurance, and all that would go out the window if Moish were forced to close up shop.

I told Moish we couldn't hold on much longer. We were losing money, and he was paying other people to do his work. To top it off, Moish was an extraordinarily honest person. If he made a mistake with a deadline, for instance, he would pay the penalty himself. That was an expensive and chaotic time for us—and I became strung out like crazy, in part because I knew that Moish couldn't apply for disability until he stopped working.

It was apparent to me that as hard as it was for Moish to sell his beloved practice, the one thing Moish was trying to hold on to, more than anything else, was his dignity. He didn't want to leave any of his clients in the lurch, but more importantly, he didn't want to tell his clients he was sick until he was sure that he could sell his practice.

It was overwhelming for Moish to try and run a practice where he could no longer do the work. I suggested that he consult with a rabbi about the situation. Although he valued my input regarding his business, I knew that my opinion alone wasn't going to sway him. Moish respected one particular rabbi, and when that rabbi told him it was time to sell his practice, Moish was willing to accept the news.

Accepting or not, it didn't change the undeniable fact that Moish and I—and by extension our family—were hemorrhaging money. I needed some clear-headed advice on the matter, so one afternoon I asked Pinky to take Moish out for the day so I could talk to Dr. Pelcovitz, a well-known and respected psychologist, about our situation.

I explained to Dr. Pelcovitz how Moish was too sick to run his business anymore. I told him how concerned I was about Moish's reputation, and how we wanted to find somebody honest—a *mensch*—who would buy Moish's practice. We also wanted to find somebody who wouldn't blame Moish for the terrible condition the practice was in.

I told Dr. Pelcovitz that I didn't want Moish to worry about whether the buyer was successful or unsuccessful. In other words, I didn't want him to feel badly if the practice fell apart or, conversely, to feel jealous if it performed well. Moish explained to me that the new owner was going to face some obstacles, because his was a service business, and many people wanted to work with Moish personally.

I was terrified that we weren't going to be able to find a buyer, and was practical enough to know that we couldn't sell the practice for what it was worth, but Dr. Pelcovitz still encouraged me to explain to potential buyers what the situation was, and to accept any reasonable offer.

Finally, after an eternity of sleepless nights, we found a woman who was willing to buy Moish's practice. She was widowed, and a mom to two lovely girls. She was looking to increase her client list. We told her that we would encourage Moish's clients to take her on, although we made it clear that we couldn't force them to. Moish's clients were going to do whatever was best for them.

Moish was very concerned for this woman, so he called his clients one by one and begged them to give her a chance. This proved to me what a good human being he was—here he was, losing a business he spent a lifetime building, and he wanted to make sure the new buyer would be okay. Moish wasn't worried that she would do a better job than him, or any of the things other people might be concerned about.

We sold the practice late in 2008 and, ultimately, the buyer and I became friends. I was grateful that Moish and I could finally get away from the practice. We both needed to be done with it.

Despite my feelings, it was hard for me to watch Moish leave because he had built his practice from nothing. It was tough, hard work, and his clients not only loved working with him, many of them had become his friends. Over time, however, those relationships dwindled. It's hard to keep a relationship up over time when you're not seeing each other day in and day out.

When Moish stopped seeing the people he worked with, he felt a loss of friendship, a loss of importance, and a loss of dignity. Somehow, throughout this transition, Moish managed to remain good-natured about everything.

With all of the unspeakable chaos going on in our lives, the *parnassa*, the livelihood, seemed insignificant to a degree—although it was hard for me to comprehend how, at this stage of our lives, we could be so broke. Still, I remember feeling that I would happily have paid somebody a few thousand dollars just not to have to meet the prospective buyers and explain to them why Moish's practice was in such disarray.

Alas, like everything else going on in my life, that was just one more thing I had to learn to cope with.

***

One of the things I enjoyed the most about working at HASC was that it took up a significant part of my time and mental energy. It enabled me, for a few hours at a time, not to dwell on Moish's sickness.

Work kept me focused, and allowed me to exist on autopilot for part of the day. I set my alarm for 5:45, and was often the first person to arrive at work. School didn't officially begin until 8:30, although it wasn't unusual for one of our kids to act out on the bus, at which point I would be called upon to intervene. On normal days, I didn't have time to prepare the feeding and medications, but on the mornings I arrived early, I had plenty of time to prepare everything, which had a calming effect on me for the rest of the day.

In contrast to my regimented workdays, the holidays became particularly dreary for me not only because my loneliness was magnified, but because I wasn't able to occupy my mind with work. I was at home twenty-four hours a day with a husband who seemed to be deteriorating before my eyes.

As much as I loved being home with Moish and the kids, there were days where I literally didn't get out of bed until the afternoon. There was nothing earth-shattering that *had* to be done so, perhaps out of self-pity, I would sometimes allow myself the luxury of bringing my computer into the bed, or a good book. I was very cognizant, during those times, how important it was for me to have something to focus on *outside* of the home. If I stayed home every day, I would begin feeling sorry for myself, and that would have a negative effect on me, on Moish, and on my kids.

***

In the Jewish tradition, it is common after a wedding for the family to celebrate the blessed occasion over the next seven nights. The entire week after the wedding is like one extended party.

Perele is Moish's only sister, and her husband is an only child; whereas Moish and I had many people in our extended family, my sister-in-law had few. Every time one of Perele's eight kids got married, I cooked for and hosted at least one of the post-wedding parties at my house. It was an overwhelming endeavor, but it was a lot of fun, and always worth the effort. Perele happily did the same for me.

During this particular feast, celebrating the wedding of Perele's sixth child, Yakokov, Moish was planning to speak—a simple, uncomplicated, fun speech that would entertain the guests. Even though Moish wasn't able to process things like he once had, he still had the ability to read and speak beautifully.

Right before he was about to stand up, Moish realized in a panic that he had lost his speech; I panicked as well, and berated myself for not having made a copy of his speech for him. Moish was constantly losing things, and I tried to make copies of anything important.

My kids and I scoured the house from top to bottom for half an hour, while Moish visibly grew more and more frustrated. My heart ached for him because he wanted so badly to feel like he was contributing to the party. Moish felt like he had let all of us down, and unfortunately, he didn't have the capacity to ad lib like he would have done in the old days.

Years earlier, he wouldn't have had to write his speech down at all.

I offered to rewrite the speech for Moish, but he was so worked up by that point that he didn't feel comfortable giving any type of speech.

"I don't feel good about myself," Moish said.

Moish was having difficulty explaining why he couldn't give a speech anymore—but truthfully, he didn't have to explain. It was obvious to me and the kids, and it was hard for us to see.

In the end, I gave the revised speech to Pinky, who did the best that he could. He and my son-in-law Dovi spoke elegantly, but I was overcome with a sick feeling in my stomach when I saw how upset Moish was.

Impulsively, I drank a full glass of wine on an empty stomach, and the whole room started to spin. I had forgotten it wasn't a good idea to drink alcohol when I was taking medication.

One of my friends saw me and gave me some water, which helped a bit. Looking around the room, I couldn't tell who else was aware of the situation with Moish and his speech.

One of my daughters said, "Ma, you look so calm. The stress isn't showing on your face like it used to."

Her comment was oddly upsetting to me. I guess I was getting better at acting cheerful when inside, my heart was breaking.

I found that with practice, I was able to put my pain on hold by telling myself I could cry into my pillow as soon as I got home. I was particularly stoic when my grandchildren were involved. I felt sad enough that they didn't have their grandfather, and I very much wanted to be the attentive, happy grandmother. When they were around I did my best to push my negative thoughts aside, although there were times when that just wasn't possible.

It generally took me about an hour to calm down when I was upset, but once I got involved with my children or grandchildren, I was able to focus on their needs. I would wait until I got home, where I would turn on some music and cry my eyes out.

***

In December of 2008, Moish and I attended a family wedding in Lakewood. We wanted to see our grandchildren dressed in their gowns and wedding outfits, but the thought of driving two hours each direction made me nervous. I had an abysmal sense of direction, and this was in the barbaric days before everybody was walking around with WAZE on their smartphones or GPS in their cars.

The wedding was beautiful; we had a wonderful time eating and drinking and socializing with our friends and family.

On our way back home, one of our acquaintances asked us for a ride home to Brooklyn. This man had some emotional issues of his own, as well as a bit of a drinking problem. I had always found him to be a bit socially awkward, but part of me felt sad for him. Strange or not, Moish and I were happy to give this man a ride, so we all headed for home in the pouring rain.

There I was with my poor sense of direction, a confused husband in the front seat, and a strange man in the back seat. To top it off, it was pouring buckets outside and I could barely see the road out the window. I was driving twenty miles an hour but still couldn't find our exit. I felt panicked, but I had to try and appear calm because the more anxious I appeared outwardly, the more upset Moish would get. I didn't want him to get nervous—especially with another passenger in the car—so I kept quiet.

All of a sudden, Moish whispered to me, "I'm not sure, but I think there's a police car behind you."

There are very few things that make a person's heart beat faster than seeing flashing blue and red lights in their rear-view mirror.

I rolled down the window and the policeman pulled up alongside of me and said, sternly, "Lady, you're in a sixty-mile-per-hour zone and you're going under twenty."

Through the rain, I pleaded with him.

"I'm lost," I told him. "I don't really know where I'm going."

"Then pull over to the right," the policeman said. "Stop blocking the traffic."

When I rolled up the window, I was taken aback to see that Moish was cackling at me. I was shaking and upset, and my husband seemed to be having the time of his life.

"You're laughing at me," I accused him.

"I'm not laughing at you," Moish insisted, although his face told a different story.

"You're loving every minute of this," I said.

Looking at my sick husband, who was practically crying from laughing so hard, I felt conflicted. On the one hand, I felt nervous and out of control and angry. On the other hand, I was happy that Moish was able to exhibit so much joy; it had been a long time since he had laughed like that.

Eventually, I found my way home. A few weeks later, during our regular visit with Dr. Horn, we told him the story. Dr. Horn seemed pleased that Moish had expressed so much outward emotion, even if it was at my expense.

***

When you're dealing with a sick spouse, there is nothing more important than your family and friends.

My brother Pinky—may he rest in peace—was the oldest of four children in our family. He had two younger brothers, and I was the only girl. We were ten years apart and had a special relationship—I considered Pinky to be almost like a father to me. He had a terrific sense of humor, and he and I had some great times together.

Pinky liked to travel. He and his family were constantly moving, and I made a point of spending half of my summers with them. When they moved to California, I went to California. When they moved to Vancouver, I went to Vancouver. I was ecstatic when Pinky finally decided to return to New York; sadly, he hadn't been living in New York long before he passed away.

When Pinky died, I truly thought I would never be happy again. Fortunately, time heals all wounds (at least to some degree), and eventually it did get easier. When Moish was diagnosed, however, I found myself missing those people—especially Pinky—who were so important to me when I was younger, and my first instinct was to reach out to him. That was impossible, but something wonderful happened. His children reached out to me. They began spending quality time with my mother, who had lived out of town most of their lives. Because of her failing eyesight, she was now joining us most weekends, and I visited her as often as possible during the week. I was essentially acting as caretaker for two people at once.

One of Pinky's daughters had ten kids of her own, but she still found the time each week to drive out to Brooklyn and take my mother out to lunch. Pinky's kids were amazing; all of my mother's grandchildren were, but there were one or two who were exceptional. I knew that when they came over to visit, I didn't have to worry about my mother.

Having Pinky's children grow close to me and my mother was like a final gift that Pinky left me. It made my mother less dependent on me, which allowed me to focus more of my attention on Moish.

I found myself thinking about Pinky a lot, and each time our family celebrated a wedding or a bar mitzvah, I really missed him. I couldn't get my brother back, but I could love him through my family.

***

I never felt the need to define it, but as Moish got progressively worse, I naturally assumed he was in the *later* stages of Lewy Body Dementia. After all, he had gone from being a funny, coherent man to a sullen, forgetful man in a little bit over two years. He was, in almost every way, completely different than the man I had married.

During one of our routine neurology visits, which often felt to me more like a therapy session, as I was able to voice my thoughts, fears, and nagging questions, Dr. Horn told me in an infuriatingly casual voice, "You do know that Moish is still in the *early stages* of this disease?"

I looked at him as if he'd told me I had cancer.

"But there's so much going on with him," I said. "If this is the early stage, how bad is it going to get later on?"

My first thought was that perhaps our doctor didn't properly comprehend how bad things with Moish were at home. My second thought was to wonder exactly how much worse this disease could possibly get.

I didn't say anything out loud because Moish was sitting next to me—and because I felt sick to my stomach.

Dr. Horn tried—and failed—to make me feel better, although his words had the opposite effect on Moish.

"In thirty years, you won't be in great shape," he told Moish with a smile, "but then again… *she* might not be either. You might even outlive her."

He pointed at me.

My mind spun, trying to imagine living this life of confusion and uncertainty for another thirty years. When I first researched Lewy Body Dementia, the average life expectancy was six to eight years from diagnosis, so the concept of enduring twenty-five more years was hard for me to grasp.

The thought of Moish outliving me wasn't comforting, although it may have been comforting to Moish, so part of me was able to feel happy for him.

CHAPTER 5

One of the main symptoms of Lewy Body Dementia is forgetfulness, and this struck Moish in a very intense manner. People often called our house during the day and left messages for me; invariably I would not get those messages, and my confused friends would ask me a few days later why I hadn't returned their calls. Then there was Moish's *daf yomi* class, which he had been teaching for eight years. He should have been able to prepare those classes easily, but the morning preparation became harder for him, and took much longer.

Over time, other "simple" things became challenging for Moish, such as reading the clock on the living room wall. Moish couldn't figure out the big hand and the little hand. He could still read numbers, so this was a quick fix—we put up a digital clock instead. This was a temporary solution, and I was terrified for the day when Moish wouldn't be able to read the digital clock either.

There was a certain level of obsessive-compulsiveness to Moish's forgetfulness. Moish had always been structured—out of necessity during tax season, undoubtedly—but he was now completely out of control. When he packed his bag for the gym, the "old Moish" would toss three or four items in his bag and rush out the door. The "new Moish" spent an hour putting the same four items in his bag and rechecking the bag a dozen times. When he wasn't rearranging things, he was losing them; I lost count of how many different pairs of goggles Moish misplaced. I couldn't get angry about this because, as with telling time, it wasn't his fault. I simply replaced the goggles. It wasn't a big deal to me, but Moish was terribly frustrated by it.

The hardest part of Moish's forgetfulness was how many of my friends thought I was exaggerating it because he looked and sounded so good. But I had the "privilege" of seeing what was going on with Moish behind the scenes, and to a lesser extent my kids did as well, although by the time he started being forgetful, only my youngest three kids still lived at home.

**

There are a million ways people have of coping with a sick spouse. Some drink alcohol, some turn to food, and some sink into a deep depression.

Me? I decided to start taking an antidepressant, which I swore my whole life I'd never take. I took it for four days and didn't feel better at all. My main reaction to the drug was that I felt like I couldn't cry, which turned out to be a good thing because I seemed to cry everywhere I went, which was getting embarrassing.

In other words, with medication I *felt* miserable, but had no tears to show for it. I told some people I had allergies—which I do have, so technically I wasn't lying—although my close friends and family knew the truth.

One person who knew the truth was my friend and former boss at HASC. On my sad days, Chaya Shaindl would take one look at me and give me a big hug. She allowed me to express my struggles and my feelings, which was a huge comfort to me, but she wasn't the only one. My co-workers at HASC touched me in many small and often comical ways. For instance, somebody read an article about how blueberries can help with dementia, so the next morning I found a large bowl of blueberries on my desk with a note: *Bring these to your husband.* Gestures like that made me smile.

One Friday night, Moish and I went to Pinky and Miri's house for Sabbath; I decided to skip my medication. The next afternoon, Miri's parents came by to say hello. The moment I saw them, I was struck by how much I missed the normalcy of a husband-and-wife relationship and the joy of marriage. At that moment, I desperately missed my previous life and my previous marriage.

I ran to the bedroom and gulped down a pill. I didn't want to cry in front of Pinky's in-laws. I needed to get my act together, or at least *look* like I had my act together, even though my heart was breaking.

***

"How come you don't talk to me anymore?" Moish asked me one afternoon. "You talk to a therapist… what about me?"

I went to see several therapists, but only Dr. Pelcowitz seemed to be correct in the advice he gave me. Dr. Pelcowitz was very busy and very well-known; normally he dealt with more traumatic situations than Moish's, but I was fortunate to be able to meet with him a handful of times.

On each occasion, he shared some brilliant insights, and talked to me in a calm, respectful manner. One of the best pieces of advice he gave me was to "tap my resources" more when taking care of Moish and my mother. For instance, he said there was no earthly reason why I couldn't ask one of my children to take my mother for an entire weekend, which would free me up to concentrate on Moish. When I told him how I was beginning to resent being stuck at home all day, he suggested that twice a month my mother should spend Shabbos with somebody else. That was music to my ears; I felt like time was running out on Moish and I being able to socialize.

As hard as it was to impose upon my children and grandchildren, I knew that having them take my mother from time to time would allow me to spend time with my husband while he was still verbal and still physically strong. Some of my nieces and nephews jumped in and hosted my mother during the holidays, which was an incredible help.

Occasionally, this went beyond my immediate family, and I swallowed my pride and asked one of my neighbors for help. If, for instance, one of my sons couldn't take Moish to synagogue, I would ask a neighbor if they would be so kind as to take him. Sometimes they were able to help me out.

Each time I saw Dr. Pelcowitz I came away feeling encouraged, although he clearly didn't have time for long-term therapy. People called on him for trauma situations, not run-of-the-mill consultations like mine.

***

In January of 2009, HASC held its annual Professional Day, at which the keynote speaker was none other than Dr. Pelcowitz himself. He gave a very nice speech about anger and happiness.

I was excited to bring Moish to Professional Day with me; I thought it was a good idea for him to see the person I had spoken about. Furthermore, Dr. Pelcowitz was a warm, helpful man, and I thought Moish would enjoy meeting him.

The one thing I remember about that day—even more than the speeches—was that everybody remarked how good Moish looked. He looked good in part because he had lost a great deal of weight; on top of that, I always tried to dress him appropriately.

After the hundreds of stories I had told about Moish, the people who worked with me at HASC were interested in meeting him in person. Many of them were shocked by how presentable he was; most of them were expecting somebody who didn't look well.

Unless they had a deep conversation—not the typical chit-chat that goes on at these kinds of events—I would venture to say that most people who hadn't met Moish weren't able to tell he was sick at all. He was definitely not the person he once was, but he knew enough to fake the small talk, and how to cover himself.

***

With Moish being so ill, I felt blessed to have four of my children—and several of my grandchildren—living close by. They were all genuinely willing to jump in and help with whatever was needed. They had good communication between themselves, and they all understood that if they couldn't reach me, it didn't always mean something was wrong; sometimes I was just having a bad day and needed some time alone.

I was grateful my children cared enough to check in on me, and that they allowed me to "disappear" from time to time without getting upset. They understood my need for space, and my desire not to appear pathetic.

I told my kids a thousand times not ever to come over because they felt sorry for me—I never wanted *anybody* to feel sorry for me. That being said, I loved their company and made it clear that if they were genuinely happy to visit, they were welcome any time.

I was not the kind of mother who guilted her kids, and even went so far as to *encourage* them to have close relationships with their in-laws. There were many times when I wasn't available to babysit, so the grandkids ended up with the in-laws. Sometimes I felt sad that I didn't have the energy to do what I used to do, but I was well aware that I couldn't do it with a full heart.

Whatever I did with my family, I wanted to do with the right spirit and attitude. If something was going to make me angry or resentful, I wouldn't do it. My children and in-law children were sensitive to this, particularly the girls, and were always quick to step in during times of emergency.

The sicker Moish became, the more desperate I became to find people who were going through the same thing I was. My mind kept returning to the amazing Alzheimer's conference I had attended, and I wanted to create something similar in my own neighborhood—specifically, I wanted to start a support group for caretaking spouses like me. My cousin David helped me place an advertisement to this effect in the *Jewish Press*.

I got a handful of calls from the ad, but not from the kind of people I was looking for. The majority of calls came from people dealing with a sick parent, which is a different situation, with different nuances, than taking care of a sick spouse. Parents are older and less mobile, whereas with an active person like Moish, you run into some very specific challenges.

One thing I found in talking with people was that some, like me, were open books, while others were surprisingly secretive about their spouse's illness.

Some people didn't even let their spouse know they were sick, which didn't make sense to me. It seemed that it could be potentially harmful *not* to tell people your spouse was sick, and it certainly didn't help to preserve your spouse's dignity. In Moish's case, the people who were mean and unpleasant to him weren't bad people—they simply didn't understand he was sick. They thought they were dealing with a man who was annoying or obnoxious, but once I explained Moish's condition to them, they invariably became kinder and gentler.

Although it was not my personal instinct to do so, I did understand why people chose to keep their spouse's sickness only among family and friends—because they didn't want to be pitied. A brain disorder like Moish's is different from cancer or similar diseases, however, because the sick person can't give you appropriate input. Perhaps they can in the beginning stages, but overall, the caretaker is the one making decisions, and the sick person is getting angry and confused with them for making those decisions.

As a caretaker, I needed support, and I needed to feel good about the decisions I was making, even when Moish got angry at me for making them.

***

When Moish was diagnosed with Lewy Body Dementia, I read everything I could get my hands on, although I dutifully tried to stick to reputable sites like the Mayo Clinic, because I never knew what was true, and what was exaggerated or downright false. At first, I ran into the trap of reading blogs where people described every single horror they were going through. I began looking for these signs in Moish, but got to the point where I could barely think straight anymore.

I consumed so much information that I became obsessed with researching Moish's disease, and I was making myself sick waiting for every symptom I read about to manifest in Moish.

Eventually, I realized that I needed to stop cold turkey. I needed to close my computer and take several deep breaths. I had enough information, and if I needed additional information in a month or two, I could easily look it up. For the time being, I simply needed to deal with the reality that had become my life.

The only person I continued to follow throughout Moish's sickness was Richard Taylor, the man I heard speak at the Alzheimer's conference. He was brilliant and optimistic but, more importantly, he himself was living with the disease. Whereas most people were advocating for the caretakers, Richard Taylor was advocating for my husband, and I loved him for it.

***

In February of 2009, Moish and I took our seven-year-old granddaughter, Suri Hellman, on a trip to Chicago to visit my daughter Malkie. Suri was very excited to go with us. Malkie's eight-year-old daughter didn't know that her cousin was coming to surprise her.

Under normal circumstances, all of the focus would have been on Suri—making sure she had the best trip of her life. Unfortunately, most of my focus had to be on Moish; his behavior and attitude would make or break this trip.

Even before Moish got sick, I was nervous and a little obsessive-compulsive about traveling. I was sure that our luggage would be lost, or that we would be late boarding the plane. My kids made fun of me because I always left for the airport hours before I needed to; they joked that we should all just go to the airport the night before. I explained to them that I'd rather be at the airport early and be calm, than rush around like a crazy lady and barely make my flight.

This flight was no different—but now instead of my own luggage, I had to take care of Suri's luggage *and* Moish's luggage, which was very stressful and overwhelming for me.

Normally, I never traveled with checked bags because it seemed like an unnecessary hassle—not to mention the potential of the airline sending my luggage to a completely different destination. On this trip, for some reason, we decided to check our luggage.

Moish, as always, was trying to be helpful. Somehow, he boarded the plane ahead of me and Suri, and without telling me, he placed one of our suitcases at the front of the plane.

When we were getting off the plane, I didn't know which piece of luggage he had put at the front, so I didn't know what I was looking for. I must have looked panicked, because Moish asked me why I was making such a big deal out of this.

Logically, I knew he was right. I knew that *I* was the crazy one in this scenario, not him. Moish was trying to be helpful, but all I was thinking was, "How am I going to manage Moish, my granddaughter, *and* all of this luggage?"

Of course, we did manage to find all of our bags in the end, but I left that airplane feeling rattled.

The luggage, unfortunately, wasn't the most stressful part of our trip. In our tradition, many Jews celebrate the one-year anniversary of a parent's death, a *yahrzeit*. This is usually observed at home by saying specific prayers, and by lighting a *yahrzeit* candle for twenty-four hours.

Without thinking about it, I had booked our flight to Chicago on the anniversary of the death of Moish's father. This meant that Moish would have to go to the synagogue in Chicago and say prayers for his father.

Moish was very worried about this. When we landed, he claimed he had only one clean shirt, even though I had packed him three. I wasn't surprised that he wore the same shirt all three days of our trip, only to find the two other shirts in his suitcase when we were safely back in New York.

On Friday afternoon, Moish went to the synagogue next to Malkie's house; not surprisingly, Moish forgot his charger and his phone died. After forty-five minutes, I called Moish to make sure everything was okay. He didn't answer. I tried a few more times, but Moish still didn't answer.

Feeling a bit nervous, I told Malkie that I needed to walk over to the synagogue and make sure Moish was okay. Moish came out and asked me what was wrong.

When I said I tried to call him several times, Moish told me that he fell asleep. Relieved, I went back to Malkie's house and let Moish stay at the synagogue for a few more hours.

Later that day, I wanted to take the girls sledding on a big hill a brief drive away. Moish didn't want me to go because he was afraid I would get hurt, but I decided to indulge my granddaughters and go.

I took the girls sledding, and we had a tremendous time. The next day we took the girls to Chuck E. Cheese, and Moish and I browsed at the bookstore. The following day Moish and I took a relatively uneventful flight back to New York.

Back in my home, I realized that I didn't want to travel with Moish anymore; it was too emotionally draining for me. From now on, I told myself, we were going to stay local.

***

Sometimes I dreamed that *I* was the one who had dementia.

This happened a few times throughout the years, although it wasn't always dementia; I was generally fearful that I would get sick along with Moish, and that my kids would be left without a functional parent. I was worried they would have to care for two sick parents instead of one. It was a very real fear of mine.

Whenever I forgot something, I tended to panic.

"Oh my G-d," I would say at work. "Am I okay?"

My co-workers laughed at me about this. One day someone told me something that resonated with my situation.

"If you lose your keys, it's okay," they said, "but if you forget what the keys are for, then you're in trouble."

I kept this thought in the back of my mind as the days wore on, and always remained on the lookout for the change.

My dreams usually reflected whatever anxieties I was feeling at the time. Sometimes I remembered them, and sometimes I didn't. Sometimes I woke up grateful to G-d that whatever I dreamed wasn't true; every so often it took me a few hours to calm down because my dream felt so real. What I found was that my dreams reflected my fears, especially if I wasn't sharing them with anybody.

***

In early March, I wrote a small note to Moish saying that it was March 4. To my great astonishment, he said, "Hey, that's our anniversary!"

Throughout our marriage, I always made a bigger production over birthdays and anniversaries than Moish did.

"Stop buying me gifts," he would joke. "Now I have to buy you gifts."

This year, I told Moish that I didn't need a gift for our anniversary, but that it would be fine if he gave me a card. Just the fact that he *remembered* our anniversary made me happy.

Moish did go out and get me a beautiful card, and he signed it himself. It showed me that he was still present on an emotional level, still had strong feelings for me, and was still able to communicate those feelings to me.

One year, Moish's sister picked out a gift and card for my birthday. When Moish gave it to me, I was devastated. When he was well, he knew that I hated to buy plants, because they would take one look at me and die. Of course, Perele had no idea about that, and bought me a plant!

I told Moish, and he must have understood because on the next occasion, he picked out a card himself. I knew the type of cards he picked out; I could tell that he had picked this one, and that made me extremely happy.

In a Judaica bookstore, Moish and I went to pick out a *sefer*, a religious book that my son Pinky wanted. Before we left I had clarified with Pinky exactly which *sefer* he wanted, but Moish insisted that it was a different one. He even picked it up and tried to buy it, but when I insisted that it wasn't the one Pinky wanted, Moish lost it.

He wanted to give this *sefer* to his son, and he accused me of making him feel terrible. He yelled at me, accusing me of not letting him do anything himself.

I tried to explain to Moish that I had just had a conversation with Pinky, that maybe he had changed his mind, but that I didn't want Moish to buy him the wrong thing. Once Moish calmed down, he understood that I wasn't trying to provoke him.

It was in situations like this where Moish's lack of short-term memory was actually a blessing. By the time we got home, Moish had forgotten that we'd had an argument. On the other hand, this argument stayed with *me* for the rest of the day. I used to feel that Moish adored me, so on the rare occasions when he was angry with me, it was hard for me to let it go.

***

In April of 2009, I was having a *terrible* day. I was late for my appointment with Dr. Pelcowitz, and in an effort to park quickly, I ended up getting a parking ticket. During the actual appointment, Dr. Pelcowitz was not in his usual pleasant mood.

To top it off, it was my birthday. I had never fixated on getting lots of gifts or spending a lot of money, but I had always liked it when people acknowledged the day. I was always careful to remember the birthdays of my friends and family—I even kept a list in my pocketbook.

After I returned from Dr. Pelcowitz', I asked Moish to take a walk with me. We went to the grocery store, and then to get him a haircut. On the way back, I told Moish gently:

"I want to tell you something so that you won't be upset tomorrow."

I started to sing "Happy Birthday," and Moish said he hadn't forgotten that tomorrow was my birthday.

"Moish," I told him. "*Today* is my birthday. I don't want anything. I just wanted you to know."

It's not about the giving… it's about the remembering. Which is why it hurt me so much that Moish completely forgot it was my birthday. Even though it wasn't his fault, I still felt upset.

Then, at the Mittleman Grocery, Shevi Mittleman gave me a bit of perspective. Shevi's husband had passed away a few years earlier, and she reminded me how nice it was simply to have a warm hand to hold.

For that, indeed, I was grateful.

***

Moish and I were never big believers in Mother's Day and Father's Day; we considered them Hallmark holidays, designed to make the card companies and the florists lots of money. Occasionally we exchanged token cards or flowers, but most years, we didn't make a big deal out of it.

That being said, on Mother's Day in 2009, I woke up with my legs feeling like lead. I was supposed to help my friend buy a gown to wear to her daughter's wedding, but I was having trouble getting out of bed and starting my day. In the old days before Moish got sick, it would have been a pleasure driving down to Crown Heights to help a friend with a fitting. But on that day, every little thing was hard for me. I literally had to talk myself out of bed, face the day with resolve, meet the challenges head-on, and force myself to smile.

At the end of that difficult day, Moish gave me two beautiful *birthday* cards.

***

When tough days arrived, I worried that I would get depressed. I'm an extremely emotional person. My girls and I joke that we're all a little bipolar—when we're happy, we're extremely happy, but when we're sad, we're down-in-the-dumps sad. I prayed that I would never experience clinical depression.

In September of 2009, I switched the medication that I was taking.

I had gained a lot of weight—which naturally didn't help my depression—so a psychologist suggested I try something else instead. It took a month or two for the new medicine to kick in, but after that I noticed a huge difference in my mood and energy level.

Once I found the correct dosage, I became a huge advocate—to the point that any time I met somebody who was feeling blue, I told them, "You know what? I have just the thing to recommend."

I know that not everybody is eager to take a pill, but if you can take something that's not going to make you sick, and that can in fact make you feel better, why not take it? I wasn't at an age where I was worried about getting pregnant, so why not?

Before I started on medication, I cried constantly, and felt out of control more often than not. The antidepressant took the edge off, which was the first step toward me feeling somewhat like my old self.

Still, some mornings I found myself fighting depression with a vengeance. There were times when I felt like crawling under my covers and sleeping the day away. Every time I tried to sleep, however, the phone seemed to ring off the hook; everyone was trying to help by arranging weekends with my mother.

I felt guilty lying under those covers. I was overwhelmed being a caretaker for two people on the weekends. I felt like a failure. I wished that I had more energy, more patience, and stronger nerves. I wished that I had what it took to be a superwoman.

All I could do was try harder.

***

As I navigated the journey of Moish's terrible sickness, I was fortunate to meet some truly inspirational people along the way. One woman, Carol, whose husband passed away after being sick with Alzheimer's for twelve years, gave me a lot of good advice, and helped me put things in perspective. One area she helped me with was when I got upset when people told me how great Moish looked. She told me that I got upset because Moish *did* look good, but that people didn't understand he looked good *because* of me. I didn't feel validated because I was the one who picked out his clothes and shoes. I was the one who brushed his hair and made sure his beard was trimmed.

Carol also lived in New York. I called her periodically to ask her questions. She seemed to understand some of the things I was having a particularly hard time with. It made me feel good to figure things out by hearing advice from somebody who had already gone through some of the same things I was going through.

One facet of our situation that I hadn't thought much about was the loss of intimacy that comes with having a sick spouse. In the Jewish law, husband and wife have to agree to a divorce, which is of course impossible in the case of severe dementia. There are times when a husband can write out a divorce agreement in advance, allowing his wife to divorce him when the time comes. This doesn't mean the wife is going to stop caring for her husband, but it gives her the freedom to marry somebody else in the future if she wants. Jewish law allows a wife to accept the divorce and remarry, which is a liberating feeling even if you never take advantage of it.

I found all of this intriguing, although it didn't apply to me. I wasn't thinking about remarrying. On the other hand, my mother remarried at the age of seventy, so anything is possible. The law can allow people to move on in the event of extremely long and catastrophic illnesses that often involve serious brain damage.

***

Moish has a first cousin named Susan. She and her husband David lived in Lawrence, about forty-five minutes from Brooklyn. Before Moish got sick, the four of us occasionally met in Manhattan for dinner. At that time Moish was seemingly working around the clock, so on the rare times he was able to go out, I generally wanted it to be the two of us. One of the few exceptions was David and Susan, who we became extremely close to.

Once Moish's sickness took him out of the picture, things became socially awkward for me with some of my friends. I felt like I was in a difficult and vulnerable position, and it affected some of my relationships.

One Friday, Susan called me at work and asked me about my plans for Shabbos. I told her that Moish and I were alone for the weekend. Susan told me she had invited Uncle Yossi and Aunt Helen, and that Moish and I were welcome to join them. I felt a little pathetic about my situation, but Moish and I went anyway. I felt that nobody else seemed to see what I did in Moish.

Moish was not the same man he once was, and I felt that every move I made was being judged by *Hashem*. That is true for all of us, I suppose, but I never felt so determined to be a pure, righteous Jew, and to do what *Hashem* expected of me.

***

Before he got sick, Moish had a tremendous sense of humor—but even after his mind began to slip, sometimes he would still purposely try to rile me up.

One day I came home from work, tired and exhausted like always. Moish took one look at me and, with a deadpan expression, said, "Excuse me... who are you?"

I assumed he was kidding, so I teased him back.

"Come on," I said. "You know who I am."

"No, seriously," Moish said. "What's your name?"

This went on for several minutes, until I could feel the color begin to drain from my face. For a moment, I had a macabre sense that this was the beginning of the end, the moment when Moish officially had no idea who I was.

Finally, Moish started to laugh. He thought this was hysterical, although I couldn't bring myself even to smile. But he thought it was funny to get my goat like that.

Moish's humor was not limited to the home front. During one of our appointments with Dr. Horn, as I was going through my long list of questions, Moish asked me: "If they find a cure for this, do I have to go back to work?"

I found that comment strangely adorable.

***

The holidays in 2009 were an incredibly peaceful time—my mother was spending time with her sister, and all of my kids were away. For the first time in a long time, it was just Moish and me. It was a cold, still night. I felt like hugging Moish and not letting him go; if I had been given one wish, I would have wished that time could stand still so I wouldn't have to face an uncertain future.

Holding Moish, I felt a slew of conflicting emotions. I used to dream fondly of this chapter of our life, when our nest was empty and we could spend meaningful, quiet time together. Once Moish became sick, I learned to treasure those times more than I once had. Every day I felt the proverbial clock ticking, and prayed that Moish would be able to continue to learn so that he could feel a purpose to his life.

During Chanukah, Moish told me he was sad that he was sick; he had always looked forward to teaching things to his grandchildren. I half-joked with him that his aspirations were more noble than mine. My dreams always focused on the two of us, going away together, taking spiritual and relaxing vacations.

"We're doing that a little bit," Moish told me, although realistically, we weren't traveling much; our financial situation kept us homebound more often than not.

I told Moish that the only thing I knew for sure was that I cherished every moment he and I spent alone together; and, ironically, that if he were well, we might have taken our health for granted and not spent as much time together as we did now.

With the kids out of the house there were fewer distractions; we were content doing simple things like listening to music and drinking hot chocolate.

One evening Moish asked me what things were going to be like when he got worse.

"I'll be here to take care of you," I assured him, "just like you would take care of me if the roles were reversed."

"Who said I would take care of you?" he asked with a smile.

I hugged him when he said that, grateful to *Hashem* that he still had a bit of humor left in him.

CHAPTER 6

Throughout our marriage, Moish was always the one who drove—which, considering my abysmal sense of direction, was fine with me. Moish never trusted me behind the wheel—and he was right not to, because half the time I didn't know where I was going. When he got sick, however, I told Moish bluntly that I didn't think it was safe for him to drive, no matter how much he wanted to. I simply didn't believe that Moish was capable of driving anymore.

Moish fought me on this, and insisted he was going to ask Dr. Horn if it was okay.

"That's a good idea," I told him, sure that the doctor and I would be on the same page.

To my surprise, Dr. Horn told Moish there was a place in New Jersey where he could take a driving test, to evaluate if he was still a safe driver.

Moish, practical even though he was sick, said, "How am I going to get there if I can't drive?"

And that, thankfully, was the end of that.

To be charitable, I told Moish that if driving was so important to him, I would take him to New Jersey—but I didn't encourage him or remind him about it, so he eventually let it go.

Sometimes I could get away with not mentioning certain things, and Moish would forget about them. He just let them be, which was more than fine with me.

Living in Brooklyn, we frequently drove to the Five Towns because some of our kids lived there. During a typical forty five-minute drive, Moish would ask me every three minutes how long until we arrived, much like a child might do.

"Are we there yet?" he'd say, over and over again.

In addition, every time we approached a stop sign, Moish asked me if I saw it... a hundred feet before. He didn't understand that I saw the stop sign as clearly as he did. Moish was so used to being the driver that for some reason it bothered him to have me behind the wheel.

I told my kids that for somebody who always sat in the front seat, Moish was a real back-seat driver.

On one trip, I got lost and found myself a little bit nervous. After having Moish ask me twenty-five times if we were there yet, and loudly announce every stop sign and stop light, I angrily pulled into a parking space and turned to face him.

"Moish," I said. "If you ask me that one more time, I think I'm going to have to kill you."

My voice was too calm for such a statement, like Nurse Ratched in *One Flew Over the Cuckoo's Nest.*

"What did you say?" Moish asked. He sounded confused and hurt.

I couldn't believe those words came out of my mouth. My voice was calm, but inside I was exploding. I did that a handful of times when Moish was in the car—I think because he made me so nervous. I felt terrible and quickly apologized.

"Just kidding," I said sheepishly.

Sometimes Moish tried to make the car cooler by turning up the radio dial. I told him that no matter how many times he turned the dial, it wasn't going to change the temperature.

I realized that was the meanest thing in the world I could have said to him, and I saw the way he recoiled. I hurt him. During those mean moments I hated myself and wished so much that I could always be the perfect wife, but on rare occasions I just lost it.

***

Moish and I preferred to lease our cars rather than buy them. When the lease was up on our current van, we leased a new Honda Accord. I felt spoiled choosing leather seats in place of the cheap vinyl ones, but I threw caution to the wind and placed the order. The salesman convinced me that, after driving a comfortable van, I should lease an equally comfortable Accord.

After emptying out the glove compartment in the old van, I joyfully drove our new car home and pulled into the driveway.

"Mazel Tov," Moish shouted; he had always enjoyed getting new cars, even more than me.

I handed him the keys.

"Do you want to drive around the block?" I asked him.

Moish shook his head. He told me morosely that he had misplaced his wallet, and therefore didn't have his driver's license.

"I just want to sit in the car," he said.

I handed Moish the keys, calmly walked into the house, and began to sob. Normally, bringing home a new car would have been an exciting moment we could share together. I felt guilty, thinking I should have leased something less extravagant, and I felt awful for Moish because he desperately wanted to drive, but his sickness simply wouldn't allow him to do so.

Many people know the popular game of dreidel, which is played by Jewish children on Chanukah. Depending on what letter the dreidel lands on, you either make money or lose money. One Chanukah, Moish bought a bag of dreidels to pass around, and he wanted to get a pocketful of change as well.

He took his twenty-dollar bill into the bank to get change for the grandkids, and came back out with… *nothing.*

Moish had given the teller his twenty-dollar bill, but didn't remember that he needed to take the change from her. I was waiting in the car, and I asked him: "How do you feel… are you sad about this?"

He shook his head in resignation. Getting proper change was just one more thing Moish had trouble doing.

I parked and went into the bank, where I explained to the very confused teller what had happened. The change was sitting untouched on the counter where Moish had left it. It occurred to me that I needed to be more watchful, because it would be extremely easy for somebody to take advantage of Moish's forgetfulness.

Things like that were painful for Moish; fortunately, his memory was getting so poor that sometimes he simply forgot whatever it was that was causing him so much pain.

Of course, whether Moish forgot or didn't forget, my heart ached for him. There was something tragic about a man who had devoted himself to the intricacies of tax law for thirty years, who now couldn't collect the simple change for a twenty-dollar bill.

One of Moish's favorite activities was going to the gym. There he could be around people and get exercise at the same time—and Moish had always enjoyed exercising.

We hired somebody to escort Moish to the gym, but on the days he wasn't able to take Moish, one of my kids would take him. On rare occasions, Moish would ride the bus by himself.

On one of the days Moish went himself, his fingerprint pass wasn't working, and the gym wanted money for a new one. He became terribly upset, and after traveling back home on the bus, his emotions were out of control. Moish thought they wanted him to pay an extra thirty dollars a month, when in reality it was only ten. In his mind, they were trying to take advantage of him.

Of course, updating his membership was something I should have taken care of, but I had so much on my plate that things like that sometimes fell through the cracks.

This incident exemplified how Moish's perceptions of things were confused. It took a concerted effort on my part to convince him that the gym was worth joining, and that he should go back.

***

Many of the things that Moish couldn't do—for instance, setting the alarm clock to go off at 6:15 in the morning instead of midnight—were annoying to me, but I tried to deal with them the best that I could. Then there were the things that made me feel sad, such as when Moish began to forget the names of his grandchildren.

At first, this wasn't particularly upsetting—or surprising— because we had so many grandchildren; there were certainly times when I struggled to remember one or the other of their names.

The first thing I noticed was that Moish forgot the names of his in-law children. He would say things casually like, "You know, Ruchi's husband… so-and-so's wife."

I never corrected Moish about this, but it was still a heart-rending moment when I realized that another stage of forgetfulness was beginning. Each time Moish hit another "milestone," I got an initial shock, after which I had to calm myself down. I was resigned to the fact that he was getting worse. First it was going to be names, but eventually he was going to forget peoples' names *and* faces.

It was like witnessing the beginning of a very depressing slope, and all I could do was pray that it would take Moish a long time to get to the next stage. Sometimes change took a long time, while other times it happened quickly.

The most frustrating aspect about this was the lack of consistency. Sometimes Moish would have a terrible day where everything seemed to go wrong, followed by two amazing days where I was almost able to pretend he wasn't sick. I woke up every day not knowing if I was going to get "coherent Moish" or "confused Moish." The more I researched Lewy Body Dementia, the more I realized that this constant shifting between good and bad days was common in people who had the disease.

I considered the good days with Moish to be a gift. They were also a reminder that I needed to be more careful on the bad days, and not assume that Moish didn't understand what people were saying. People sometimes came into our home and talked to Moish like he wasn't there; even I was guilty of this on occasion.

The painful thing was that the good days started coming less frequently. On those good days, I felt like dancing I was so happy. It pleased me more than anything when Moish was aware—even temporarily—of what was happening around him.

***

Although Moish was forgetful and had very little short-term memory, he still tried to accomplish certain tasks—it just meant that when he did, things sometimes ended badly.

One afternoon he and I went to the hardware store. Moish asked one of the workers where he could find the Ice Melt, and she directed him to aisle five.

Since Moish didn't have any memory, by the time he turned around he wasn't sure if the Ice Melt was on aisle five or six. This type of thing happened on a regular basis. The saddest part about it was that sometimes Moish *would* remember things, but his memory was generally so poor that people didn't believe him, even when he was right.

I went to aisle five, while Moish went to aisle six. Moish began calling me, and by the time I found him, he was completely exasperated. I couldn't tell if he was upset because he didn't remember what aisle the worker had told him or because he couldn't find me, which frightened him.

We eventually found the Ice Melt, but Moish was complaining that the worker had given him the wrong information.

This type of situation presented me with a dilemma—trying to find a balance between Moish's independence and his frustration when that independence backfired on him. I wanted to let Moish do the things he wanted to do, but I also knew that if something proved too difficult for him, Moish was going to feel worse about himself.

As bad as Moish's short-term memory was, I was grateful that his long-term memory was, at least for now, very sharp, meaning that visits from people who knew us long ago were pleasurable, because Moish seemed to remember many stories from his past.

Sometimes Moish's forgetfulness was humorous. There was one time when we couldn't find our cordless phone. We searched all over our house, pushing the finder button, trying to get it to ring.

Instead of listening for the tone, however, Moish kept picking up the other phone and saying hello, which of course meant we weren't able to find the one we were looking for.

I told Moish that if he kept answering the phone, we were never going to find the other phone. He didn't have any idea what I was talking about. This went on three or four times, until finally I told him we would just leave the other phone where it was.

Things like that were so ridiculous that I could laugh hysterically at them, or else cry like a baby about them. Part of it, for me, came down to accepting the fact that losing and finding things was simply going to become a big part of our lives.

Moish *was* able to follow simple directions, but only one at a time. Doing anything became a tedious step-by-step process. For instance, if Moish was making hamburgers, I'd have to tell him to open the refrigerator, then take out the hamburger buns, then turn on the stove, then put a hamburger on the stove, and so on.

Then there was the chaos that resulted from his forgetfulness. For instance, on more than one occasion I found an article of clothing in the refrigerator. There were other things—some of which, admittedly, were issues before his sickness hit—like remembering to put the seat down on the toilet. When I asked Moish to put the seat down now, he told me he preferred it up.

I had to make a conscious effort *not* to make things like these an issue—if Moish wanted to keep the seat up, was that really the end of the world?

I learned an interesting lesson about dementia from Moish's father, who developed the disease in his eighties. I remember one time coming to pick him up; he forgot that I was coming, and he asked me if I had called to tell him I was coming. I said yes, and I could tell by his face that I'd make a huge mistake. He was mortified when he realized how bad his memory was; I learned this lesson when it came to dealing with Moish.

I never made it seem like Moish had repeated a question, even if he had asked the same one a dozen times. That was harder than it sounds; there are times when it's pure torture to answer the same question over and over and over again.

I became good at keeping a straight face, and equally good at not bringing needless things to Moish's attention. There wasn't anything to be gained by "setting him straight." It was hard enough for him to live like he was living—pointing out every mistake he made would have been cruel.

***

Resentment is an inevitable emotion in a situation like mine—not all the time, but it's bound to come up here and there.

One thing I resented was people giving me advice that I didn't ask for, especially when I only saw them once or twice a year.

One time somebody asked me, "Have you ever considered bringing some movies to show your husband?"

I wanted to yell at them, "Are you kidding me? I have thought of every single thing imaginable... every single thing! If it's not out here on display, it's because it didn't work!"

I had gone out and bought a dozen movies I thought Moish might like—old-time movies like *The Three Stooges*. When they didn't work, or Moish didn't respond to them, I'd move on to the next thing. I tried everything I could think of to keep him occupied.

I wasn't vicious or unkind to people's faces, because I've undoubtedly made hurtful comments to other people without realizing it.

There was a certain child at work who laughed a lot, and I thought he might be having seizures, so I wrote what I intended to be a helpful note to his parents. As soon as I got the answer back, I knew that I had unknowingly aggravated his mom, who had already researched her son's diagnosis to death. Her response to my letter was, in effect, "I've been dealing with this situation for over ten years, so I think I know best."

I could tell instantly by her tone that I had overstepped my bounds, and it made me realize that most people mean well; sometimes things just come out of our mouths. In this instance, I called up this parent and apologized. Fortunately, she knew that I had good intentions, so there was no lasting harm done.

***

In the Jewish culture, the *machzor* is the prayer book that is used on the High Holy Days—Rosh Hashanah and Yom Kippur. In our neighborhood, on the occasion when one of the High Holy Days fell on a Saturday, we didn't carry things.

Before the holiday, I wanted to bring the prayer books over to the synagogue. I handed Moish three prayer books—one for me, one for Moish, and one for our friend Sondra, who was staying with us during the holidays.

Moish couldn't remember what I had said, so I took away all of the *machzorim* except three. I told him to take the top one for himself and to put the other two by my seat. He came back in a few minutes and told me he needed another *machzor* for himself. I told him he had already brought one for himself, so he tried again. But no matter how many times I sent Moish across the street, he kept getting mixed up. Finally, my mother said, "Why don't you go with him?"

I went across the street and found the two *machzorim* on my seat.

"I don't know where my *machzor* is," Moish said.

"Check your seat," I said.

"It's not there," he insisted.

"Check your locker," I suggested.

Moish checked his locker and grinned.

"It's here," he said… and then proceeded to put the *machzor* back in his locker.

"Tonight is Rosh Hashanah," I said. "You need to take the *machzor* out because you're going to use it tonight."

"Tonight is Rosh Hashanah?" he asked.

"Yes," I said. "It's both Shabbos and the first night of Rosh Hashanah."

Moish was surprised, but he took his *machzor* to his seat.

That night, I told my mother that she had given me good advice to go to Shul with Moish—but I felt sick to my stomach as I did so.

I badly wanted Moish to have some semblance of independence, but in cases like this, sometimes it seemed ridiculous that I didn't go and help him. Little things like this had become unbearably complicated, and they certainly got me in the spirit of crying in prayer. By itself, it wasn't a big deal at all—but when twenty similar things happened in the course of a few days, I found my delicate balance crumbling. I had to remind myself that when I, or other people, told Moish something, there was a good chance he wouldn't remember it in the least.

***

Moish was always very strict about keeping kosher. There are different levels of keeping kosher; the rules are extremely complicated, and everybody has their own way. One of the things that Moish did that I wasn't so strict about was only buying bread and cake that had been cooked by a Jewish baker.

I have always liked a piece of coffee cake on Saturday morning, even if I'm on a diet; it goes perfectly with my morning cup of coffee. One Friday I was working, so I asked Moish to go to the store and grab some cake—but Moish forgot.

Moish had picked up some food at Meisner's take-out, but I had forgotten to give him a list. I told him to get a *challah*, a few rolls, and some cake. When I returned home from work, I saw that Moish forgot the rolls and only bought a tiny piece of cake; he told me he returned some of the cake because it tasted old and he didn't know what to buy.

When I realized we didn't have cake for the morning, most of the stores were already closed, so I told Moish I would run over to Key Food and find something. I found a package of Stella D'oro cookies, which is something Moish didn't eat, but which I loved.

Moish made a comment to me, "So, now you're eating Stella D'oro cookies?"

I lost it, and in a rage, I dumped all the cookies in the garbage and left the house in a downpour. I walked for blocks and blocks, allowing the raindrops and tears to drip down my nose.

When I returned, I took a hot shower, made two cups of hot cocoa, and brought them up to our bedroom for Moish and for me.

"You're the one who didn't get the cake to begin with, so get off my back about the Stella D'oro cookies," I explained to him. "I want a piece of cake with my coffee in the morning, and I'm eating them."

As I was speaking those words, I was thinking to myself, "Hennie, you're insane. Who cares about cookies and cake—it's such a stupid thing to get upset about."

Once in a while, I lost my mind over something trivial—I tried hard to let so many things go. It seemed like sometimes the smallest thing was the straw that broke the camel's back.

Moish never imposed things on me when he was well. He acted differently once he became sick, but sometimes I couldn't help reacting badly. Moish probably was just questioning me because I didn't usually buy that brand of cookies.

After I explained to Moish about the cookies, he told me that when he shopped, he needed an exact list. Just being told to buy cake was too overwhelming.

Moish also said that he was insecure.

"Wow," I said. "You're insecure and I'm depressed."

"It should be the other way around," he said.

I told Moish that I was having trouble dealing with day-to-day life, and I needed him not to criticize me.

As we sat there drinking our cocoa, I began to think about all those people who deal with mental illness, and how absolutely horrible that must be for their families.

***

One of the symptoms of Moish's disease was that he had vivid auditory hallucinations.

Sometimes, out of the blue, he would ask me, "Did you hear that?"

"I didn't hear anything," I would say.

"Listen!" he would say, often looking frightened.

When I researched this, I learned that people with Lewy Body Dementia often have auditory hallucinations, when they hear things that aren't there—simple things like a toilet flushing.

At one point, Moish's hallucinations were getting bad, and waking him up in the middle of the night. It was frightening for him… and for me. I never argued with Moish about what he was hearing—I was sure it sounded real in his mind.

I discussed this with two different doctors, and they both told me that taking Klonopin would help him. Once Moish started taking that medication, the hallucinations lessened considerably, and Moish was definitely calmer.

One less thing I had to worry about, with the help of Klonopin.

One down, I thought, five hundred to go.

At the same time, Moish's daily paranoia began to get increasingly out of hand. One incident in particular made it clear to me—and to others—that Moish truly was not in his right mind.

My brother Hertzie assisted me financially on more than one occasion, and often did things I would not have been able to do. In one instance, he took my son Yitzi to the Apple store and bought him a three hundred-dollar iPad.

It so happened that Yitzi was traveling to Israel, so Hertzie asked him if he could take a toy to one of his grandsons who lived there. My son happily agreed—after all, what harm could there possibly be in it?

Moish, however, thought there could be *tremendous* harm in this.

"You can't take people's things," Moish insisted. "Don't you know that people hide *drugs* in these toys?"

We couldn't help smiling, and Moish noticed.

"You're laughing at me," he said, "but you heard about the boy over in Japan. There was a big incident, and a kid got caught. Somebody messed him over; it wasn't his fault."

Moish was not making this story up, and in fact it was well-known in our community. A Jewish teenager carried a suitcase full of drugs into Japan without knowing it; somebody told him they would pay for his plane ticket if he carried their suitcase. The teenager was naïve, but he went through hell for that one mistake. His story was in all the papers, and was a big deal in our community.

"I do know the story," I assured Moish. "I do know that people have drugs, but we're talking about my brother here… he's not going to put drugs into a toy for his grandchild."

Moish couldn't tell the difference between the two cases, which meant that his judgment was impaired—and it was this type of thing that other people had so much difficulty seeing.

***

Having a sick husband, I witnessed several people who were rude and uncompassionate toward Moish. They were a thorn in my side every time I encountered them… but thankfully, they were balanced out by people who truly knew how to demonstrate compassion and empathy.

One of the nice things about our neighborhood in Brooklyn was that we lived close to everything we needed—grocery stores, busses, trains. We didn't need a car, which was convenient for Moish. Several people in the neighborhood knew Moish, making shopping easier for him. People were happy and willing to help him out.

One day Moish went into Schwartz's Appetizing store to buy a few items. One of the men who worked there was a man who prayed in the same synagogue as Moish. He was in the back, but he overheard Moish at the front counter, having difficulty figuring out how much to pay.

This man came running out to the front and told the cashier he would take care of Moish. That was a blessing for my husband, because he understood that he was having problems, and that this wonderful man was helping him to save his dignity.

Moish was grateful that he was able to go to a store without being humiliated. And I was grateful that Moish was able to come home and repeat the story to me.

I knew the man Moish was talking about, and I regret that I never told him how much his small actions meant to me.

Having a sick spouse also made me ultra-sensitive to how other people treated *their* sick spouses.

Moish and I were sitting in the lobby, waiting for one of his myriad neurology appointments. There was only one other couple in the room, and it frightened me to see a person who was further along than Moish in their disease progression. I was able to see, depressingly so, what my future might look like.

The wife, who was the sick half of the couple, was asking her husband what year it was.

"You're kidding," he said, in a snide, hurtful tone. "I can't believe you're asking me that. I just *can't believe* you're asking me that."

I'm sure that my mouth fell open. How could somebody not understand a situation that was undoubtedly occurring on a daily basis? I wanted to go over to the husband and explain, "She's asking you because she doesn't know the answer."

It was obvious, from his words and his body language, that he hadn't yet accepted that his wife was sick.

I was struck then and there that having a sick spouse required a true act of acceptance; you need to get to a point where the person's actions don't strike you as strange. If they ask you a question, they're genuinely curious about something, and you owe it to them to answer... with gentleness and empathy.

In this case, although I desperately wanted to confront this husband, I kept my mouth shut; it simply wasn't my place to say anything about it.

I felt terrible for the woman who was sick, knowing that her husband's attitude was most likely not an isolated incident. Although it didn't reach that level, it made me think of the cases of elder abuse that seem to be so frequent. The husband couldn't acknowledge that his wife had a sickness; he simply thought she was being annoying. It was similar to those instances when people didn't have patience with Moish, although it's infinitely sadder when it's somebody's spouse.

***

When Moish was first diagnosed, I didn't feel angry at all. At the beginning of Moish's sickness I was prepared to take on his challenge with full force. Sometimes I felt lonely and sad, but surprisingly, I still felt extremely close to G-d. I was in a very secure place with my religion, and was confident that G-d was going to protect me.

My attitude was bolstered by my children, who were amazing to me and their father—and to each other—throughout this whole process. They were my most important blessing and support during a very dark time.

Other than my children, I also turned to books for solace. I read dozens of books when Moish was first diagnosed, but was surprised by the level of anger that some of the authors seemed to have. I would think it would be the people who were sick who would be angry, as they were the ones missing out on a significant part of their lives—but sometimes the caretakers seemed to be the angriest.

I simply couldn't comprehend how I could be angry if Moish wasn't.

***

Many of my days with Moish blended together, while others in particular stood out.

One Friday night, I was alone with only Moish and my mother. It happened to be one of the Friday nights where Moish was stricken with his terrible abdominal pain. On this instance, like it often did, his pain was accompanied by bouts of nausea, and he threw up several times.

My mother spent most of the time downstairs, as walking up the stairs was difficult for her. On this night, I was trying to have a pleasant Sabbath conversation with her, but every fifteen minutes we'd hear the horrible sound of Moish vomiting upstairs.

I interrupted our conversation three or four times until Moish calmed down and was able to get to sleep, but by then we had both lost our appetites. Each time I came down the stairs, my mother looked so pitifully sad.

"I don't think I can do this," she told me.

My mother needed me, but very seldom did she have my full attention. My attention was primarily with Moish, and that made my mother feel lonely. She needed somebody who could focus on *her* needs, and I simply couldn't be that somebody for her.

Thankfully, it was around that time that people began inviting my mother over for the weekend, which was a huge blessing for me because it allowed me to concentrate on Moish guilt-free.

CHAPTER 7

In 2010, I set out to write an article about my experiences as a caretaker. This stemmed from my disappointment a couple of years earlier when I attempted—but failed—to start a support group for spouses affected by dementia.

I kept asking myself, "What else can I possibly do to reach people?"

I concluded that writing an article in a popular Jewish magazine might be a possibility—I thought that if it got printed, perhaps people would reach out to me. I became excited at this prospect, although several of my kids were tentative about the idea.

One of them told me, "We're not exactly keeping a secret here, but writing an article is like making a public announcement."

I thought long and hard about what my kids said, and in confusion I turned to my cousin David, who gave me sound advice when facing a dilemma like this.

"My kids aren't thrilled with this idea," I told him, "but I really want to write this article. What do you think I should do?"

"Call them back," he said, "and tell them that you know they're not excited about you writing an article, but that it's something very important for you to do. Tell them that you're asking for their blessing, not their opinion."

I did what David suggested, and it worked like a charm. Every one of my eight children said something to the effect of, "If you need to do this for yourself, go for it."

Of course, I knew that my kids were having all sorts of side conversations, but I didn't care. To me, they were very gracious and supportive about it.

I submitted my article to a Jewish magazine called *Mishpacha*, a weekly publication with a quarter-million readers. I wrote a few drafts with my sister-in-law Lolly's help, although my kids encouraged me to write future articles in my own voice.

I couldn't believe how many people read my article and called to congratulate me on it. I heard from people who knew me well, and from people I hadn't talked to in a long time. Overall the response was extremely positive, and I was able to find a small silver lining amid the horrible situation I was living in.

Not only did many people read my article, I even received an invitation for a speaking engagement, which made me extremely happy.

Once I published that first article, I felt compelled to write others... and I did. The first article was definitely the most exciting, and I felt a tremendous sense of accomplishment about it.

I'm not sure that Moish was completely cognizant about what I was doing, although he knew that I liked to write in my journal. By the time the article was published in early 2010, however, he wasn't aware enough to understand it; this was opposed to 2008, when Moish and I read several books and then discussed them. Moish read "Still Alice" and told me that it was very realistic, and that he could relate to it. We also enjoyed "Alzheimer's From the Inside Out" by Richard Taylor.

***

From the time he had his first memory lapse, I worried that one day Moish was going to get lost in our neighborhood— after all, every so often you hear a story on the evening news about a dementia patient wandering away from their house and getting lost in the woods for several days.

What if the same thing happened to Moish?

What if he got out of bed while I was sleeping and walked right out of our house?

What if I couldn't find him?

During one of our neurology appointments, Dr. Horn tried to convince me to give Moish more freedom than I was giving him, so I told him about my fears.

"You live in a safe neighborhood," Dr. Horn insisted. "Let your husband have his freedom. He has his phone if he needs it."

I looked morosely over at Moish; he was wearing his phone holder, but the phone itself was nowhere to be seen. When Dr. Horn noticed this, I could tell what he was thinking.

The phone's not going to be much help if it's not on him.

I asked Dr. Horn if there was some sort of medical bracelet Moish could wear, something that would allow people to contact me—or the hospital—if he got lost.

As much peace of mind as that would have given me, part of me *didn't* want Moish to wear a bracelet, because it felt like I would be announcing his sickness to the world. I didn't think that everybody needed to be aware of the bracelet in every situation.

Doctor Horn, on the other hand, thought it would be a smart idea. He told me it didn't have to include too much information—just my telephone number along with a note like "Allergic to Ativan" or "Memory problems."

One problem with the medic-alert bracelet was that Moish was unable to get it on and off by himself. It had to be tight enough so he couldn't slip it off his wrist, but even I had a hard time removing it with both hands.

One night a friend of ours visited us. For some reason we began talking about medical bracelets, and he pulled out a medical necklace I didn't even realize he was wearing.

"Look at this, he said. "It's comfortable, it doesn't bother me, and it's not where everybody can see it. If it needs to be out there, it is, but I can also just tuck it in."

It was simple. It was brilliant. It would be easy for Moish to take off over his head. And we could write whatever we wanted on it. Using the necklace would be a very simple solution to our problem, and I found myself very excited about it.

The whole "bracelet versus necklace" conversation pointed to a larger issue—when I would stop allowing Moish to go out on his own. I went to work every day, and I worried that he was going to get lost in his own neighborhood. This thought was nerve-wracking to me, and I found myself second-guessing myself.

Was I being overprotective? Was I being underprotective? This was a tough balance for me, because I knew that if anything happened to Moish while I was away, I would ultimately be the one to blame.

The same thing applied to physical tasks, such as allowing Moish to ride a bike when I knew he might fall. He *did* fall once or twice, but the bike gave him a huge feeling of independence. That, and the ability to exercise outdoors in the fresh air, far outweighed getting one or two scratches. Of course, I would have felt differently had he broken his leg or gotten a concussion, but I did take chances with certain things and, praise G-d, most of the time it worked out okay.

***

In 2010, my daughter Ruchi gave birth to a baby boy, so at the end of April Moish and I prepared to attend the bris (the circumcision). We drove out to Far Rockaway the night before, so we could help watch the grandkids the morning of the bris.

As I instinctively drove into the EZ Pass lane, I realized I had left my EZ Pass in the old van. A surly police officer immediately stormed out of the ticket booth and began yelling at me. He told me I could be subject to a summons and a ticket—and that I was blocking traffic to boot.

I rolled down my window.

"I'm sorry," I told the officer. "We just leased a new car and I left my EZ Pass in the old car by mistake."

"So, you didn't notice that you were sitting in a new car?" the officer said sarcastically. "Show me your license."

I began to get rattled, and couldn't find my license. I started ripping apart my entire pocketbook while Moish tried to calm me down.

"Take your time," Moish said. "It's going to be okay."

The unpleasant officer continued standing at my window, glaring at me, waiting for me to explain.

I turned to him with tears in my eyes.

"Can I tell you something," I said. "This probably won't mean anything to you, but somebody in my family is really sick, and my head isn't working too well."

The officer's countenance changed instantly.

"I *can* understand that," he said. "I really can; I'm sorry to hear that. Why don't you just pull over there and give me two-fifty."

I practically had a heart attack.

"Two hundred and fifty dollars?" I said. "For going in the wrong lane?"

"No, two dollars and fifty cents," he said.

I reached back into my purse and gave the officer his money. As I did so, I wondered what he would say if he knew that the sick family member I was referring to was the man sitting so calmly next to me. Still shaking, Moish and I drove away.

A few days after that incident, I retrieved my EZ Pass and decided to call and see if I could use it in my new car. That should have been an easy transaction, but the phone number they had on file was the old one from Moish's office in Brooklyn. When I said I couldn't remember that one, they asked for the last four digits of his credit card. Moish had replaced his card, so he didn't have that either. The bottom line, since we had a new license plate, was that we had to apply for a brand new EZ Pass.

I hung up the phone, exasperated at how complicated things seemed to be getting these days.

***

Moish had a very kind heart, but sometimes his kindness unintentionally backfired.

On one occasion I sent him to the ice cream store with some of our grandkids—how much damage could he do there?

The first thing that happened was that Dovid, my grandson who was allergic to nuts, came back holding a cup of ice cream, telling me it was a Coffee Coolata, which was the only thing in the place that was safe for him to have.

It definitely didn't look like a Coffee Coolata; it looked like ice cream, which could have given him an anaphylactic reaction. Thank G-d he hadn't taken a bite yet.

The second thing that happened was I asked Moish to bring home two extra quarts of ice cream—but he arrived with five. I thought I had only given him enough money for two quarts, so I was concerned that maybe he had taken some ice cream he shouldn't have.

When Moish went back to check, the manager said they were making some new flavors and he gave them to Moish for free.

In theory, that was very generous of them. In reality, however, I wanted them to stop being so nice. All it did was confuse Moish and when he got confused, I got confused, which then made all of our lives unbearable.

It never occurred to me that maybe the "mistake" didn't have anything to do with Moish. I finally settled down and focused on the fact that everybody had their ice cream, that Moish was happy because he was spending time with his grandchildren, and that nobody had eaten anything that required a trip to the emergency room.

***

It took Moish a long time to get dressed in the morning— thank G-d he still had his sense of humor. One morning he told me that by the time he got his pants on, it was going to be Rosh Chodesh again—the beginning of the new month.

Moish's spine began to curve as a result of the Lewy Body; he shrank two or three inches, meaning that some of his pants were suddenly too long. Moish told me that soon he and Uncle Yossi, who was five feet at the most, would be the same size.

That reminded me of a joke my uncle used to say: "I used to be very tall, but my wife cut me down to size."

***

Although Moish had many rough days, every so often he had a delightfully good day.

Moish and I were running errands on Avenue J, and Moish had been so confused lately that I began to feel depressed. To compound things, when we walked out of the shops I completely forgot where I had parked the car. Because of my terrible sense of direction, I used to rely on Moish to get me where I needed to go. But he was as hopeless as I was, except for today.

I started to look for my car, feeling frustrated and confused, when Moish said, matter-of-factly, "You're going the wrong way; you parked the car over there."

Normally when he said something like that my instinct was to ignore him, but today, something made me trust him. He took me by the arm and led me directly to our car.

I was ecstatic—not just that I had found my car, but that Moish was given a rare opportunity to help. It was apparent to me in those moments that there were times where Moish *could* think clearly. There wasn't any rhyme or reason *when* these moments came about, but I certainly appreciated them when they did.

I took advantage of his good days by calling my kids.

"Tati's having a good day," I told them. "Try to come over today, even if you were planning on coming tomorrow. I don't know what things are going to be like tomorrow."

***

Shortly after the EZ Pass incident, my kids threw a sixtieth birthday party for Moish. Everybody came out—all the kids and grandchildren, Moish's sister, and my mother. Moish had a beautiful, amazing time.

We held the party at our house—we set up bounce houses for the grandkids in the backyard. It was fun watching Moish so excited, jumping on the bounce houses with his grandkids. We bought fried chicken, had a wonderful photographer, and set up the Wii—Moish loved playing the Wii with his grandkids. Moish was laughing his head off the whole time.

The whole day was extremely special; I still have a photo album devoted to that one party; we even managed to get a family picture with everyone in it, which was a miracle. Moish's party was a huge event and it meant a lot to him… and to me.

CHAPTER 8

We've all heard the famous baseball expression, "And the hits just keep on coming…"

There were days when I felt the same way about Moish. He began having a really hard time with daily tasks, and it seemed like these came about one after another after another.

For instance, Moish was always an avid reader, but he began to start books and not finish them, something he had never done before. He needed to be reminded about basic things, like which day was Shabbos. One day Moish wore an old hat out in public, and I realized he couldn't distinguish the old hat from a new one. The hat he was wearing was one that our grandkids used to play dress-up; feeling rather sad, I threw it out.

Small tasks were becoming noticeably more difficult for Moish—and not just mentally. Not only did I need to repeat instructions several times, his coordination and dexterity seemed to be diminishing as well.

Moish was living in the present, but his perceptions were severely off. When Moish fell asleep, he often existed in a semi-conscious state, somewhere between being awake and falling asleep.

Each day with Moish presented its own challenges, and I knew that my job as his caretaker was to try and face each of those challenges head-on.

One weekday afternoon, I needed to mail a gift to Malkie at the Mail Hut, the kind of place where they package everything for you. The Mail Hut wasn't far from where we lived, but it was on a notoriously busy street where the police seemingly ticketed everybody who parked there. If you wanted to do business on that street, the only way was to double-park; although if the police caught you doing that, they might *still* give you a ticket.

I knew that Moish wasn't capable of mailing the package, but in my desperation, I asked him to go inside the Mail Hut and bring out the piece of paper I needed to fill out—the UPS form with the address on it. I double parked while Moish ran in and out, hoping the police wouldn't notice me.

The street was crawling with cops, and Moish was nervous that I would get a ticket, but he reluctantly agreed to grab the UPS form for me.

I sat in the car, sweating and worried. I knew that if I stayed put I was in danger of getting a ticket. On the other hand, if I drove around the block again, Moish would never be able to find me. I decided to chance the drive around the block—as I drove, I pictured Moish coming out in a conniption because he couldn't find my car. I began having a full-blown panic attack, thinking, "Why did I think this was a good idea; why did I trust Moish to go into the store?"

Furthermore, I knew that Moish would have to come out of the store ten times to ask me questions (Is the value over $100? Do they live on California Street or California Avenue?), which he did. Each time I answered his question, I sent him back into the Mail Hut, and continued driving around the block, thinking, "I'm going to lose him; he's going to wander off somewhere, and I'll never find him in this crazy neighborhood."

I knew I was going to have to stop doing things like that because I couldn't handle it emotionally. I wanted Moish to be able to run into a store and do an errand for me without coming out a dozen times, but I knew it had to be in a quiet neighborhood where there was plenty of parking. When we were in a chaotic situation like this, I got riled up, which then got Moish riled up.

Eventually, after answering all of his questions, I asked Moish to go back and pay. He told me he wasn't sure if he had any money, although I knew he did. He then told me he had lost his phone, but it was there in the car.

Finally, after circling the block another time or two, Moish came back with the receipt in hand, his mission successfully accomplished. He did exactly what I asked him to do, but for some reason I felt like I was going to burst a blood vessel.

On another afternoon I sent Moish to the grocery store; that was one of those times when I unknowingly gave Moish more independence than he could handle. I left a simple list of items for Moish to pick up at the grocery store, and faxed a list of things for the grocery store to deliver. I also left a check for Moish to use at the store; I meant for him to give the grocer the check and pay the rest in cash.

On his way to the grocery store, Moish called me at work.

"I need to pay for the grocery delivery," he said, "and I have your list."

"What list do you have?" I asked him.

He read me the fax I had sent to the grocery store.

"Moish, I left you a different list," I said. "Do you have it?"

"No," I said. "I'll go home and find it."

"Let me give it to you now so you don't have to go back home," I said.

Moish told me that he didn't have a paper or a pen, so I simply told him what we needed.

"Buy whatever you want, and I'll get in touch with the grocery store later," I told him.

When I got home that afternoon, I noticed we were missing most of the things on my list—a dozen eggs, milk, and Danishes. I sent Moish back to the grocery store with another list, and miraculously he brought home the right things—although it did require two phone calls from the store.

While that was a fairly minor incident in the grand scheme of things, it was an example of the craziness that went on all day long.

***

In order to stay physically healthy, Moish began going to the Jewish Community Center twice a week to use the treadmill and to swim (after taking an hour to pack his bag for this excursion). Normally I had somebody drive him to the JCC, and he rode the bus home. Although Moish seemed to have trouble with the bus route, he always managed to get home. Taking the bus was one of those situations in which I tried to give Moish some semblance of independence, even though I still worried whenever he went out by himself.

Things began to get noticeably harder for Moish—and not just getting dressed or packing for the gym. He began to falter even having "normal" conversations. He began to forget commonplace names, and also the names of the people he was talking about. Moish often seemed aware of how things were going for him, but I couldn't tell exactly how clearly he saw the "big picture" of his condition. No matter how bad things got, however, I always tried to make Moish feel secure and loved—unfortunately, that wasn't always as easy as it sounds.

On one afternoon I dropped Moish off at the house, but realized that he didn't remember the combination to the front door even though I had written it down for him many times. I parked in front of the house and waited to see what would happen.

The paper never seemed to end up where he could find it, so on that day I wrote the combination on an index card. Moish took the card and put it in his wallet.

"Don't put the card away," I told him. "You need to look at it so you can open the door."

"You didn't give me a card," Moish said.

"Let me see your wallet for a minute," I said.

Moish handed me his wallet. I took out the card he had just put in there.

"This is the combination for the front door," I said. "You need to use it to open the front door."

"Okay," he said, and then proceeded to put the card in his wallet again.

I tried to stay calm, but my teeth were clenched.

"Moish, take the card out and take it with you to the front door," I said.

Moish managed to do this—I waited until he got inside the front door, and only then was I able to drive away. Thank G-d that Moish wasn't able to see my tears.

It was bad enough that Moish couldn't get in the front door, but it was even worse when he started going *out* the front door at all hours of the day and night.

Moish often mixed up his days and nights and started to wander, which naturally worried me to death. What if we were both sleeping, and Moish got up and walked out the front door? That thought literally kept me up at night until Zevi came up with a brilliant solution.

We had three locks on our front door, all of which Moish could open. We also had a combination lock because on the Sabbath, we didn't carry extra things like keys, so instead we could just punch in the combination and turn the lock.

All of our family knew the combination and let themselves in.

"We can turn the combination inside out," Zevi suggested, "and then Tati won't be able to open it because he'll never remember what it is. The only bad thing is that if you don't lock the other locks, anybody could walk in the house because it's open."

Most of the time the other locks were closed, so we tried Zevi's idea and it worked brilliantly. The interesting thing was that Moish didn't have this issue with the back door; for some reason, he always walked out the front door.

One nice side effect of Zevi's plan was that it didn't hurt Moish's feelings—he would simply try to open the door and wouldn't be able to get out. Then he would forget about trying to open it and go on with his day.

***

During one of our appointments with Dr. Horn, he told us that Moish had done poorly on his most recent neurological exam, and was therefore eligible to take part in a clinical trial. The trial was supposed to be a two-year study in which they would give Moish either new medication (which inhibited the enzyme that generated the plaque) or a placebo.

My main concern about the clinical trial was that it would be harmful to him—maybe they would give him some promising new medication but it would make him sick. Every few months I asked the doctors, "Anything hopeful regarding a cure for Lewy Body?"

"Not yet," was their inevitable reply.

There was a lot of advertising out there that made it sound like there were some cures in the works, but nothing that made me feel truly hopeful. Regarding the trial, I simply didn't know how many tests, and how many different medications, they were going to put Moish through.

One of the things they needed was a stool sample. They sent me a complicated, fancy-looking contraption, and explained that they needed me to collect the sample at a particular time. The problem was, the time they gave me was when I was at work.

I gave Moish two options—either he could call me when he needed to use the bathroom, or he could wait until Friday and I would take a day off from work. Moish felt terrible about this; he was obsessed with taking care of this as soon as possible. On Thursday morning, he called me and told me it was time to do the stool culture. One of my colleagues covered my shift for one hour, and I attempted to run home and collect the sample with the futuristic-looking gadget they had given us.

I followed the directions the best I could, which were nonsensical and bizarre. I prepared the culture to have Moish take it to Columbia on the subway. Thankfully, Perele offered to drive him. I thought that was the end of it, but that evening the doctor called and told me I had to try again because, for whatever reason, the sample I sent wasn't acceptable.

I had lost a day of work sending the incorrect sample, and I asked if I could have a couple of days to collect a new one. But the doctor told me they needed it right away. I learned, to my chagrin, that the people in charge of the trial weren't concerned whether or not I was at work—they needed things when they needed things, and they certainly weren't going to bend over backwards to accommodate *my* schedule.

The next time, we managed to collect a sample that was acceptable to the doctors at Columbia. So much for fancy stool cultures, I thought; let's bring back the old-fashioned ones and we can all get on with our lives.

***

The clinical trial involved more than just medicine; there were nearly a dozen other tests involved—MRIs, EKGs, blood tests, and interviews. I knew it was going to be difficult for me while I was working, shuttling Moish to all those different appointments, but I was willing to do it. I had Zevi talk to a rabbi, and he came back and said, "Go for it. Give it a shot… you never know what's going to happen." I found that I was actually excited about this, and so was Moish.

For the most part, the tests weren't so bad, although at first Moish was frightened of having an MRI. He eventually figured out that if someone kept touching his hand or leg when he was in the machine, he was less claustrophobic, because he knew someone was right there by his side.

After a week or two of these tests, Moish was ready to start taking the medication. My neurologist called me from Japan and told me that Moish could not be on one of his current medications, Dilantin, and still remain in the study. Ironically, for quite some time I thought that Moish should be weaned off Dilantin, a seizure medication with myriad side effects, and for months I had been asking the doctor about it.

"Why would you tamper with it?" the doctor asked. "Moish isn't having seizures. He's looking good. He's healthy."

Now, suddenly, this same doctor was telling me he couldn't be on the medication. I felt that Moish needed a seizure medication of some kind, either the old one or a new one. The doctor suggested that he try a new anti-seizure medication, but he wanted to give it simultaneously with the medicine (or placebo) from the clinical trial. Although Moish did not have a seizure disorder like epilepsy, seizures were sometimes a by-product of dementia and neurodegenerative disease.

The problem was that if Moish suddenly fell ill or had any side effects, we wouldn't know whether it was a result of the new seizure medication or the test medication. I told the doctor I needed to think about that for a few days.

As I debated what to do, another question popped into my head.

"Let's say this test drug actually works," I asked the doctor. "Suppose you find something, and Moish gets better. Am I then going to have access to that drug?"

The doctor gave a long pause before he answered.

"You could be part of another study," he said.

In other words, the answer was no, I wasn't going to have access even if it worked.

I decided I was done—the two factors together were too much to handle. It would be bad enough not knowing what was causing negative side effects if there were any, but it would be flat-out devastating to find a medication that worked, and not be given access to it.

The doctor was disappointed with me, but I didn't care. I didn't ask any questions this time. I didn't talk with my kids or with any rabbis. I just lifted up my hands and said, "I'm done... *we're* done." I didn't want any part of it.

Admittedly, part of me felt a little bit bad, because perhaps I was turning my back on some miracle cure—but I haven't heard anything about it in the time since, so I guess it didn't amount to anything.

***

On one snowy Shabbos, Moish and I bundled up and walked to Perry and Daniel's house for lunch. On the way, Moish slipped *three separate times*. I caught him, thank G-d, but on the way back home, Moish slipped and skinned his knee. Nothing was broken; he only ripped his pants and had a raw spot on his knee, but that was the first time I realized that not only was Moish fading mentally, his physical balance and dexterity were getting worse as well. It was snowing, which didn't help, but

Moish was noticeably less steady on his feet than he used to be—which gave me something new to worry about.

One thing that Moish's sickness did was force me to try and stay one step ahead of his illness. For instance, once I saw that Moish was having trouble walking, I immediately began researching wheelchairs, because I knew he would need one in the future. A few years later, I went through the same process and purchased a stairlift for him while he was still able to climb the stairs.

Moish's balance wasn't particularly good, so as a precaution I took him to the optometrist to have his eyes checked. When the optometrist told me that Moish's eyes were fine, I considered that *bad* news. If Moish's eyes were great and he was still falling, it was his balance and depth perception that were the issue. Moish was tripping over things because he didn't see them; something was not registering correctly in his brain.

The funny thing was, the optometrist thought he was giving me good news, when in fact I would have been thrilled if it had been "bad news." If Moish's issues could have been solved with a simple prescription for eyeglasses, that would have been the best news ever.

***

Many times when our kids came to visit Moish, I was home. One of my daughters, Miriam, lived an hour away from us. She had several young kids, so naturally she had to work around their schedules. Most times when she visited, she brought her youngest baby with her.

One afternoon, Miriam decided to visit her father on a day I was at work. She spent several hours visiting with him, and she told me afterwards that spending time *alone* with Moish made her realize how much I compensated for his losses.

Miriam realized how difficult everything was for Moish, and how sick he really was. She wanted to take a walk with him, and it took half an hour just to find a jacket for him to wear. By the time Miriam finished her visit and drove home, she was crying because it was the first time she recognized how clearly impaired Moish was.

I knew that I frequently compensated for Moish, and that it often masked the extent of his illness to other people. For instance, if we were out together and he didn't know who people were, he was friendly and could "get away with it," but when he was on his own, he wasn't able to function as well.

***

Despite everything I was going through with Moish, I still went to work every day—often feeling sad and guilty. I felt guilty that I didn't have dementia, guilty that my life was full and my days were busy, and guilty that Moish's daily existence was often boring and lonely.

As Moish became increasingly limited, many of the hours between his planned activities were interminably boring. We tried to get people to come over and visit, and we tried taking him to the gym, but Moish had always been a person who filled every minute of every day, beginning early in the morning.

I was now micromanaging his life. I went to work with people I loved and my life was busy and fulfilling, while Moish simply waited all day for me to come home. Every day when I left for work I felt like crying; when I walked through the door at the end of the day, Moish's face looked like a sad puppy.

For a short time, I told myself that maybe I should stop working. I thought that maybe I should stay home full-time, but I knew deep down that I couldn't do that. I didn't have the patience to be a caretaker around the clock. There were a number of years where I was the sole caretaker at night… it was just Moish and me. We didn't have help, but that was okay because I had my own space during the day.

If I had been with Moish day *and* night, I would have gone crazy. Still, I constantly felt guilty because he was stuck with minimal things to do and I was so busy.

Moish and I were fortunate that some of our kids lived close. They visited him often, although it wasn't the same relationship as before. They weren't seeking their father's advice like they used to. Instead, it was more of a caretaking role for them, which gave them a great sense of loss.

Moish and I lived very different lives, but one thing we did have in common was our near-constant exhaustion and desire to sleep. He was exhausted from his disease and from the medications he was required to take, while I was exhausted by the constant worrisome thoughts that occupied my head.

***

At a certain point, I felt that perhaps it wasn't completely safe for me to go to work. Although I had people checking up on Moish throughout the day, I still felt like I was taking a risk. My kids and some of the neighbors looked in on him, but we didn't have a steady person I could rely on.

It was a difficult situation for me because I knew that Moish needed help, but he wasn't at the point where he *knew* he needed help, so it was hurtful to him.

This was different than when Moish left his job; it wasn't a "rip off the band-aid" situation; it was one that I wanted to ease Moish into so he didn't feel judged or demeaned.

I had a friend who occasionally took care of elderly people, and I asked if she knew of anybody who could spend time with Moish in a way that wouldn't get on his nerves. I didn't want a hired person from an agency, but more like a friend.

My friend told me about a man named Yossi, who was one of her son's friends. He was looking for some type of work, and she suggested that he might be interested. When she called him, it turned out he *was* interested, and when I met him I liked him immediately. He was young, vibrant, and excited about the prospect of spending time with my husband.

My only dilemma was how to approach Moish about this. I invited Yossi over for a meal on Shabbat; we often had guests over for the Sabbath, so it didn't seem unusual.

Yossi came and proved to be very pleasant; he and Moish seemed to forge an instant connection, and I was going to delicately mention that Yossi was looking for work, and that maybe it would be a good idea if he came and "hung out" with Moish at home, and took him on errands—to the gym, or to the store, or to the library.

Before I even had a chance to say anything, however, Moish got a big smirk on his face and began waggling his finger at me.

"I know what you're doing," Moish said.

"What am I doing?" I said, as innocently as possible.

"You invited this man to our table because you want him to stay with me," Moish said. "You want him to watch me and take care of me."

Everybody at the table held their breath, waiting for some sort of explosion.

I felt trapped—what could I say to diffuse the situation?

"You got me," I admitted to Moish. "You're brilliant. That's exactly the truth."

"I don't feel like I need anybody," Moish said. "Do you think things are so bad that all I can do is stick labels on cans?"

"Of course not," I said, "but I'm nervous about you, and I would feel better if you had somebody here with you."

To my great surprise, Moish said, "Okay, we'll try him out."

I arranged a schedule where Yossi would come over and spend time with Moish when I was at work. At first, Moish seemed fine with Yossi, who was smart and personable. For reasons I never understood, Moish eventually became resistant to Yossi, and even became angry when he came over.

After a few months of this arrangement, I had to take Yossi aside.

"It's terrible, because we like you so much," I told him, "but we don't know what's setting Moish off. I can't spend every day at work knowing that my husband is angry and upset."

It was a difficult decision for me, but ultimately, I had to let Yossi go.

***

I was blessed to have some truly helpful people in my life—perhaps none more so than Zevi's mother-in-law, Malka Fass. She ran an agency for in-home health aides, and knew a lot of people and had a lot of pull.

I needed help day and night, because I still wanted to work and have a life—but Moish was also awake quite a bit at night. I needed a decent night's sleep so that I could go to work the next day. I would have hired aides, but it would have been extremely costly to hire people for twelve-hour shifts, since I would be paying them by the hour.

What Medicare initially offered was to provide a single aide who would do a twenty-four-hour shift, which wasn't good because that person would sleep eight to ten hours a night in Moish's room. That wasn't going to help me.

I was ready to give up, and I told Malka that I couldn't fight anymore. I told her that I would just settle for one twelve-hour shift and stay home myself the rest of the time.

"You're not going to do that," Malka told me bluntly. "We're going to battle this to the end."

I got turned down by Medicaid each time that I appealed for two twelve-hour shifts, but Malka was right—if you just keep on fighting, often they will give you what you want. I thought that Medicare might agree to give me another three or four hours—but I was both shocked and elated when they gave me the entire twelve-hour night shift.

I felt extremely lucky, but I didn't talk much about it because I knew so many people who were dealing with the same issue. I felt guilty for my good fortune because now I could spend whatever time I desired with Moish. I could sleep when I needed to sleep, which was a true gift.

As I lay in bed, I praised *Hashem* for sending me somebody like Malka Fass, who worked so tirelessly to get me the best and most comprehensive help she could.

***

One of the things people don't immediately think of when their spouse gets sick is all the financial and legal documents they have to deal with. I learned quickly that it was important to get help from people who are experts in different fields, because the amount of paperwork required is enough to make anybody go crazy. It is important not only to fill the paperwork out correctly—which is easier said than done—but in a timely manner. People get in trouble when they wait too long; one missed deadline can mean a logistical or financial nightmare for *years*.

The most important expert I consulted, in my personal situation, was the Medicare/Medicaid expert at Senior Care, who thankfully was familiar with the laws in New York. The reason he was so important to me was because there was no way I could function without health aides, and because I wasn't going to get any health aides for Moish—even with Malka Fass' help—without filling out reams of paperwork.

They kept torturing me, sending me more and more paperwork. One time I sent over one hundred pages from

Moish's medical report, and they told me I was approved. They couldn't believe it when they read what Moish had gone through.

The second most important thing I did was talk to an estate lawyer to figure out how to switch all of our assets—which consisted mostly of our house—into my name. This was important because in some cases, in order to qualify for Medicaid, everything has to be in your name; the person who is sick cannot have assets in their name.

I also filled out a healthcare proxy, giving me the power to make decisions for Moish. Then, of course, there was writing a will for Moish, which I put off longer than I should have.

All of those things were emotional for me—but unfortunately, they were a necessary evil in a situation like mine. For one of the experts, I made two separate appointments. I went to the first appointment alone; this was the one where I had them explain exactly *what* I was signing, and *why* I was signing. Once I was confident in what I was doing, I brought Moish along to the second appointment. He had no problem signing paperwork, so I made sure it was always conducted in a proper and dignified manner.

***

Sometimes Moish acted aggressive, which became hard for me to manage. I don't know if it was because he didn't know who I was at the time, but there were certain incidents where he grabbed me a little bit too hard—either out of frustration or because he was upset. It hurt physically, but it hurt even more emotionally.

Moish also slapped one of his health aides once or twice, although unlike me, they were able to laugh it off. I didn't find this type of behavior one bit amusing, and I told myself that we needed to find some sort of medicine to make him calmer.

Seeing Moish act aggressively was unsettling because it was so much out of his character.

Fortunately, after some trial and error, we were able to find something that settled Moish down—a mixture of Clozaril and Klonopin. Once we adjusted the dosage, Moish became calm. People used to tell me their sick husbands became aggressive and agitated at times, and the doctors would tell them it was simply a by-product of the disease. I didn't buy this; I was never going to accept that being aggressive was simply part of the disease.

My thought was, it might be "part of" the disease, but that didn't mean we couldn't mitigate it. No matter how sick or confused somebody might get, no matter how far gone in their dementia they are, there is always something that can make them feel a little bit better. I was never willing to give up hope and accept the fact that I was stuck with aggressive behavior. I was willing to go through every medication there was until I found one that helped Moish to stay calm.

Moish wasn't able to communicate his needs. I tried many things that didn't work. Looking back, I think that perhaps Moish was actually having gallstones, which were extremely painful. I had no clue, and I certainly didn't want to put him through an unnecessary surgery—but when it happened a second time I knew we had to go through with the surgery.

I was very grateful when Moish had his gallbladder out. He was a very different person after that surgery.

Although Moish's aggressiveness was hard to handle, every so often something would flip in his brain and he would kiss my hand. It was during those times that my husband's beautiful, heartwarming smile simply melted my heart.

CHAPTER 9

In October of 2011 I invited several of my family members over to our home for the Feast of Tabernacles, or *Sukkot*. That would have been a stressful undertaking even without a sick husband; thankfully, Moish now had his three aides who came in and helped him around the clock with everyday tasks such as getting dressed, going to the bathroom, and showering.

Unfortunately, right before our guests arrived, we discovered that Moish's room was infested with bedbugs, although they seemed to be contained to his room, praise *Hashem*.

I called my son-in-law, who worked in nursing homes at the time, for any bedbug advice he might have. He suggested getting a dog that could sniff the whole house and determine if we had bedbugs anywhere else. After the dog, my son-in-law told me we needed to fight the bugs either with chemicals or with heat.

Initially, the dogs determined that the bedbugs were only in Moish's room. I approached the topic delicately with all three of Moish's aides and offered to pay to have the dogs sniff out any potential bugs at their houses. I said that they couldn't come back to work unless they were sure that their own homes were bug-free.

The aides were understandably upset, and all three refused to have a dog brought into their homes. Rather than accept my offer, they all quit, and I was suddenly stuck taking care of Moish by myself. Not knowing what to do, I threw everything out of Moish's room—all the sheets, the chair, everything.

Now, in addition to a nasty infestation of bedbugs, I had nobody to help me with my husband and a house full of company about to land on my doorstep.

My only recourse was to attack the situation with a sense of humor, so I bought my houseguests little pins with bugs on them; we all wore them in honor of the bedbugs.

My son-in-law hired a company to blow heat into all of the rooms in our house so the bedbugs would be killed, which was fine, but what I didn't know was that I would still have to wash all of the linen in my house, and that I would still have to deal with all the dead bugs. It was a huge undertaking, and when all was said and done, I *still* found a live bug in the linen closet next to Moish's bed.

I went crazy, even though I knew that one bug didn't necessarily mean the entire house was infected. What worried me more than the bugs were the aides. They were excellent, and I didn't want to lose them.

Pinky called and asked them to come back.

"My mother loves you," he pleaded, "and you know she's a good person."

Two of the aides agreed to come back—and the new replacement for the third aide was phenomenal.

I didn't want to bring the bedbug issue up with them again, but one of the aides did tell me she chemically cleaned her whole house top to bottom. The other one told me that her superintendent insisted there were no bedbugs to be found in her building.

I believed them both. I hired them back and everything worked out. All in all, it was a very difficult holiday for us.

In order to comfortably house all of my guests, Moish and I temporarily moved downstairs to the office; this allowed us to give one of our kids the upstairs bedroom, which afforded them privacy they otherwise wouldn't have had.

While I was okay with this temporary arrangement, Moish seemed upset by it. He didn't react well to change, and I had to balance making life easier for my kids versus making life harder for my husband. I was torn—I knew that moving Moish downstairs was turning him into a nervous wreck. It wasn't just the change of bedroom; having all sorts of people in the house made the day-to-day routine more stressful for Moish, which in turn made it more stressful for me.

***

In the summer of 2011, Moish began to exhibit symptoms that mirrored Parkinson's Disease—shaking of the limbs, tremors, stiffness, and a general feeling of unsteadiness. Seeing Moish physically unable to navigate his surroundings was painful, but it wasn't as painful as the dementia.

Moish's physical limitations didn't change our lives as drastically as his mental ones—until he couldn't sit in the stair lift. That was complicated because I didn't have another way to get him up and down the stairs. I didn't want to move him downstairs permanently, because I thought that the bathroom situation made it undignified. Moish had lost the ability to care for his personal functions, and I didn't want to turn my house into a nursing home. Upstairs, his room was right next to the bathroom, which was very convenient.

Moish's physical deterioration was difficult to watch, but it was nothing compared to the pain I felt when he stopped recognizing me and our kids. It was at that point that I realized I had lost my best friend.

I wasn't able to have a real conversation with Moish anymore, and he had always been my go-to person for everything. Early on in our marriage, my mother-in-law would tease me and say, "You know, you don't have to tell your husband everything… it's not the end of the world."

I laughed at her and thought, *But I do have to tell Moish everything.*

Moish and I had a very honest and open marriage—maybe I wouldn't immediately mention something that I knew might upset him, but eventually it was going to come out. I was born with a guilty conscience. I couldn't live with myself keeping secrets, and I always insisted that our marriage be rooted in complete trust of one another.

As horrible as Moish's mental deterioration was, it did allow me to take on the role of caretaker, as opposed to the role of spouse. In many respects it was easier. I didn't have to consult with Moish in order to make him feel involved. I didn't have to act like everything was the same between us, because it wasn't.

Suddenly, people understood the situation. Moish had a vacant expression on his face, and rarely said a sentence that people understood; in the past, people thought he knew what he was talking about, even when he didn't. At this point, people could clearly see that he was confused.

On rare occasions, of course, Moish *did* know what he was saying, but the words simply came out wrong. I found the irony of that to be extremely sad and depressing.

***

Also during that summer, I went to visit a new doctor, Dr. Gold, who worked at Mt. Sinai. I was prepared to hate him—I had a chip on my shoulder when it came to meeting new doctors, but I walked away feeling impressed. One of the things I liked the best was his willingness to communicate via email; that was something that had long frustrated me about some of the other doctors.

Doctor Gold was very warm, and he made things more bearable for me. I no longer felt alone, as I knew he was only a quick email away. He helped me navigate some of my most difficult periods by helpfully analyzing what I told him, and adjusting Moish's medication to meet both of our needs. For instance, he prescribed Seroquel and Klonopin to combat Moish's loss of control and his psychosis.

Although Dr. Gold graciously replied to my emails, he eventually got sick of me; maybe I was more annoying than I thought I was, but I was determined to be a fierce advocate for my husband, and a busy doctor like him was going to have a hard time appreciating somebody like me.

***

I used to be very confident about the decisions I made. Even when we were first married, I could make quick decisions, while Moish took an inordinately long time making them. If he went to the store to buy a suit, he'd go in and out three times before selecting the one he wanted. I could walk in and decide in ten minutes which suit he should choose.

When Moish became sick, I began second-guessing some of my decisions—especially when they involved Moish. I started to become insecure about my decisions, and would ask other people for their input. I started listening to other people, and questioning myself much more.

In the past when I asked Moish his opinion about something, he would sometimes say teasingly: "What's wrong with you… since when do you need another opinion?"

Of course, Moish did make many of the big decisions in our life—such as moving to Israel for three years—but I was persuasive, quick, and stubborn, and I think that often Moish gave in to me.

Once he got sick, everything changed, and I suddenly felt like I was the indecisive captain of a sinking ship.

***

Not long after we made the switch to Dr. Gold, Moish had a seizure on his way out of the synagogue. It was right across the street from our house, and he must have fallen down. Fortunately, there were lots of medical personnel on our block and in our building, so they arrived on the street the moment he fell.

Zevi was with Moish at the time, so he ran across the street to get me.

At this point I was in the mindset that I was *done* with hospitals, because I knew what to do when somebody had a seizure. I had a medication called Diastat that I knew would work; if I hadn't had that, I would have had no choice but to drive Moish to the emergency room. But I *did* have the medication, and I knew there was nothing else they could do for him at the hospital. The man from the ambulance insisted I was making a terrible mistake, and Zevi told me that I should go to the hospital to be on the safe side, so I gave in and let the ambulance take him.

This happened on a Saturday, which made things difficult. Even on the Sabbath, I could do things like ride in the ambulance with Moish. But I wasn't able to turn on the television, which meant I would be sitting in a dismal hospital room until sundown, with a person who was sleeping off their seizure. All the while, I knew that there was absolutely nothing the doctors and nurses could do, and that it would pass, and that Moish would be fine.

I didn't know what caused Moish's seizure, although I did know it was unusual. Occasionally, when people with dementia have a seizure, it's because they need a medication dose adjustment. As horrible as the word "seizure" sounds to most people, they didn't usually frighten me because I worked with kids who had seizure disorders. If you can't get the seizure to stop, that's when it becomes an urgent medical situation; but if the seizure does stop, like it did for Moish, they can simply sleep it off. Although I knew that being in the hospital wouldn't do Moish any good, I wasn't secure enough to fight with everybody.

While the seizure per se didn't frighten me, I did notice a bit of a deterioration in Moish after the incident. I just didn't know if the seizure itself *caused* his downhill slide. Moish didn't seem as healthy afterwards. On the other hand, maybe I was being abnormally paranoid and neurotic, reading into every little thing he did.

On top of his seizures, Moish had some terrible bouts of constipation. This is a common problem in people with brain damage, primarily because they're not moving around as much as other people. No matter how much medication Moish took, it always seemed to be a recurring problem.

There was a child at HASC who had a full-blown seizure, the first one she ever had at school. When I spoke to her mother about it, she told me that one of the things that had caused her seizures in the past was extreme constipation. Over the years, different parents told me different things that caused their kids' seizures; I filed them away in the back of my mind and would subconsciously be on alert for them. In the end, it took a lot of effort on my part to help regulate Moish's bowel movements, but like all of us it made a huge difference in how he felt physically. It amazed me that constipation could make a person so sick as to end up with an emergency hospital visit.

***

Moish's anxiety rose to such a horrendous level that he literally was unable to sleep. He spent an exhausting stretch of four straight days where he took only very short naps.

I was forced to get aggressive with Dr. Gold's office, and insisted I was bringing Moish in. The nurse on the phone told me they didn't have any available appointments, but I told her I was coming anyway.

I was very stern with the nurse, which is against my nature. Finally, after going around in circles, the doctor picked up the phone, and although I sounded calm, I was hysterical on the inside.

"I'm very worried; Moish isn't sleeping," I explained, "and he's not moving his bowels."

"Sounds like he needs to be hospitalized," the doctor admitted.

I was relieved to hear that; I was worried that Moish might actually die from lack of sleep. Although the doctor consented to bring Moish in, it was at that point I realized that he didn't really have the time or energy to be invested in Moish's care. That realization was one of the low points of my life.

It turned out to be one of the worst weeks of Moish's life, too. He was acting completely psychotic, and I would have thought that with all of that staff, Moish would be safe in the hospital—but I learned that they followed a completely different set of rules for people with dementia.

Everything was a battle.

At first, they put Moish in a room with four beds, even though I knew that no other patient would be able to tolerate his behavior for more than twenty minutes. Furthermore, Moish needed a quiet and calm environment.

"Don't worry," the nurses told me. "*All* the patients in that room are confused."

That's when a miracle happened.

There was a man in our neighborhood—a friend of Pinky's—named Boruch Ber Bender, who was constantly doing good deeds for people. I don't know how he did it, but somehow, he arranged for Moish to have a private room at the hospital—which is what he really needed.

Moish's new room had two doors that locked behind him, although they didn't really need to lock the doors, since one of my kids or Perele and I were both in the room with him.

Even in a private room, Moish wasn't able to relax for a minute. He thrashed about, and although he desperately needed sleep, he wasn't able to calm down long enough to do that.

He was as agitated as I'd ever seen him.

The nurses said they were going to give Moish a sedative and take him downstairs for a CT scan. My daughter Perry, who is also a nurse, and I were doubtful about their ability to do that, but we didn't protest.

When we arrived downstairs, Moish started to scream and stand up on the stretcher. The imaging technician instructed us to take him back to his room and not to bring him back until he was sedated.

Perry and I knew that wasn't likely to happen, but the technician didn't believe that.

The next day we tried again, with similar results. I knew I wouldn't consent to a third try, but I also kept wondering, "Is Moish the first person with dementia to have a CT scan? How come nobody has a clue how to do this?"

Perry and I returned to Moish's room, completely drained. I requested that the nurses give him Klonopin, but they didn't seem to understand how bad Moish was. They had no sense of urgency at all, so as a last resort I opened both of the doors. I was *done* trying to explain what was going on in that room.

Moish ran out of the room in his pajamas and socks, past the nurses' station in the middle of the room; he ran in circles, hitting the walls and being completely aggressive, as the nurses were screaming, "He can't be here without shoes—he's going to fall!"

Thankfully, my kids took turns staying with me at the hospital. My daughter-in-law Lizzy explained that she put Moish's shoes on three separate times, but each time Moish kicked them off.

Moish continued to act crazy until, finally, my requested dose of Klonopin arrived.

I realized that the staff simply didn't know how to handle Moish. They weren't with him day in and day out like I was, so they couldn't comprehend the severity of the situation.

Once he took off running, however, they began to understand. The medicine began to work, and Moish was just about asleep when a friendly young man from housekeeping came in and said he had to clean the floor.

I begged him not to clean the floor at that moment because if he woke Moish, it might take *hours* to get him back asleep. I tried to explain this without making the cleaner upset. He was a little bit limited and a little bit frightened; he kept coming into the room and begging me to let him wash the floor.

"They're going to blame me," he pleaded. "I'm going to get into trouble."

"We appreciate you so much," I assured him, "and if anyone files a complaint I'm going to explain that it's completely my fault. I'll explain that I was the one who sent you out."

The man didn't look entirely convinced.

"We're not going to be able to leave this hospital until my husband is able to sleep," I explained, "and he just fell asleep five minutes ago. If we wake him up now, we're going to have to stay an extra day or two in the hospital. I'm begging you to wait a couple of hours, and then you can come back. If you can't come back it's okay; I'm going to tell everyone that you came in to wash the floor, and that I sent you away."

At that point, the man calmed down, and he wished me well and left.

Throughout this entire ordeal, I only saw Dr. Gold for a total of about five minutes. He didn't seem "present" with Moish, and mainly seemed annoyed with me. Admittedly I asked a lot of questions, and maybe I *was* a bit annoying, but he simply didn't understand what I'd been going through all these years, but especially this past difficult week. Even my aides, who were patient as saints, told me that things were out of control.

It was at that point that I decided to go back to Dr. Horn. Dr. Gold simply didn't have time for us—and I rationalized that even if I couldn't reach Dr. Horn, at least I liked him. He didn't act like I was an inconvenience or a bother.

In certain circumstances, he even went above and beyond. For instance, when Moish had his gallbladder out at Mt. Sinai, Dr. Horn came over to make sure that Moish was safe. Usually gallbladder patients stay in the hospital a single night, but Dr. Horn felt it would be better for Moish to stay two, to make sure his mental status wasn't affected. I dropped Dr. Gold immediately after that.

***

After a few difficult days, it came time to check Moish out of the hospital—but even that didn't go smoothly.

It was pouring outside when we were discharged, and the hospital lobby was overflowing. Pinky went to get the car and bring it to the front.

I could tell that Moish felt uncomfortable in that lobby; he was sensitive to noise and crowds, and quickly became overwhelmed by new people and places.

There was a guard at the door, a sullen, unruly looking man who walked over to me.

"There's a seat over there for your husband," he said.

"Thank you," I said as politely as possible, "but he won't sit."

Moish was on lots of medication, and was wobbling like he was going to fall on the floor. The other people in the lobby were staring at this disheveled-looking man with the unsteady gait, who I was holding on to for dear life. Moish was making quite a scene.

The guard began to get angry with me.

"I told you there's a seat over there," he said. "What's wrong with you? People are staring."

"Don't you think that if I could get him to sit down, I would?" I told the guard. "He doesn't want to sit."

It was like talking to a brick wall. The man didn't understand at all.

"What do you mean?" he said. "Just make him sit down."

"He won't sit," I insisted.

The guard continued telling me about how if Moish fell, there would be a lawsuit against the hospital. He showed no compassion at all, and I realized that the people who understand dementia completely are those who deal with it on a personal level.

Fortunately, the guard didn't force the issue—although he kept scowling at us until Pinky brought the car around.

It was frightening to take Moish home in that condition. I had to take care of something around the corner for a minute or two, and I remember thinking how dumb it was of me to leave Moish alone even for a few minutes. Anything could have happened to him in that short amount of time.

***

Living with Moish, I developed a better understanding of how to relate to people with brain damage. I also learned that it is impossible to know how much a person with brain damage understands.

Because of my horrible experience at the hospital—and of how generally misunderstood I felt by so many people—I became more sensitive at work, so much so that one week at our staff meeting I asked if I could give a speech about my husband. I related it to the situation we faced at HASC. I tried to imagine what we as staff members could do to help those parents who were going through so much.

I told my co-workers that we didn't need to call the parents every single time their child was having a bad day—it was hurtful for them to hear. These parents needed a break sometimes, and it would be helpful to call them when their child was having a *good* day.

We needed to focus on the positive, not just the negative.

I told my colleagues to imagine what our parents felt like every time their phone rang. They braced themselves for some awful news, but then that anxiousness turned to glee when the news turned out to be good.

As a school, we tried to be good about this. It lasted for a while, but then wore off, like those things do. Personally, I tried to keep up with it. If a parent had a smartphone, I would try to send them pictures of their child smiling or laughing or dancing; I could only imagine how wonderful that made them feel.

Living with Moish on a daily basis made me realize how important it is to learn to communicate with people who are mentally challenged. There is a language that everybody understands. That is unconditional love—showing you care by willingly and selflessly giving away a few minutes of your time.

At HASC, of course, I wasn't there for a few minutes—I was there for hours at a time. I was able to observe how even the lowest-functioning kids reacted to certain stimuli.

For instance, we had a sick child who was also blind. She couldn't move, but she knew the voices of her teacher, and when she heard it she would laugh. It was extremely sweet and touching to see.

There were other kids who responded to certain types of music, and still others who didn't "look" smart, but who in fact understood everything we were saying. I remember one child who was working with words on index cards, and he created entire sentences out of those cards. Nobody watching him would have believed he was capable of that.

We also had savants—the type of kids who never forgot a phone number or a birthday. There was one kid who knew everybody's license plate—he even told me when my registration was due.

The bottom line was, between Moish and the kids at HASC, I developed a sensitivity to how people categorized other people.

I wasn't the only member of my family who became more sensitive. Zevi told me about how he was driving down the street and saw a man—whom he immediately classified as a "raving lunatic"—running in the middle of the street.

Before his father got sick, Zevi would probably have called 9-1-1 and driven past—which is understandable, as most of us would be too scared to stop if a person looked really out of it. But Zevi understood the man's pain. He pulled his car over, stepped outside, and tried to approach the man slowly and talk to him in a calm, reassuring way. He put his arm around the man and said, "Let me help you."

"Please help me," the man yelled. He was clearly freaking out, but didn't know how to ask for help.

Zevi didn't know whether it was dementia, or psychosis, or mental illness, but he brought the man to a safe spot and was able to get help for him.

Hearing Zevi tell that story helped me to realize that nobody goes through something for nothing. Everything we go through is for a reason, and I feel that my family members have become very sensitive to people with dementia, so much so that they seem to identify these people everyplace they go.

Watching people with dementia—including Moish—it often shocks me how frequently their clarity comes and goes. I have watched Moish put his head down and sob with frustration. I have seen children at HASC who can't talk, but who then cry at their graduations. I've watched children with severe brain damage vocalize with music.

With lots of these people, it's almost like a curtain going up and down. You never know when the clarity will appear or, conversely, when it will go away. The more I live with Moish, the more I realize how little I know.

Hashem runs the world, and every day is a miracle. But as long as there is life, we need to show our love and concern for those people who don't have the gift of clear communication.

***

Several months before my youngest son, Yitzi, became engaged, Moish regressed terribly. He became psychotic, paranoid, and extremely anxious. He didn't remember his children's names, and often forgot who I was, or when I was there.

My son Yitzi was in Israel with some friends. He saw a girl on the street, and told his friends he was going to marry her.

Yitzi thought she was the most amazing girl he had ever seen. He reached out to her, and they started dating.

When Yitzi came back from studying in Israel, he brought her over to meet me. My concern, as Yitzi's mother, was that they should know each other well and both be on the same page.

In the next few months they became engaged, and I became overly stressed. I put the engagement party—which, in another state of mind, I would have loved to throw—in the hands of my son and daughter-in-law, Zevi and Devora. I knew I couldn't handle it, but they graciously made the arrangements for the party. I paid for it, but they did everything else.

Before the party, Moish was sitting quietly in the living room. He wasn't saying anything; we were nervous that he was going to get upset because of all the people, and all the loud noises. Moish didn't like commotion. He even used to shush Norma, one of his aides, because Moish thought she talked too loud.

We didn't know if Moish knew that Yitzi was engaged; he hadn't called any of his children by their correct names in months. He recognized them as his children, but he didn't have the names to address them.

An hour or so before we were going to get dressed for the party, we decided that somebody should stay home with Moish. It seemed too overwhelming—for Moish and for us—to bring him. I felt bad that we couldn't take him, but I knew in my gut it was the right decision.

All of a sudden, without warning, Moish stood up out of his chair and said one word.

"Yitzi."

My son turned around in astonishment. His father hadn't spoken his name in months. Moish walked over to Yitzi and put his arms around him.

"I just want to congratulate you," Moish said.

It was an amazing moment. Yitzi was bawling; we were all in awe, because we didn't know that Moish knew. He just couldn't tell us he knew until now. It took so much effort to speak that single sentence that Moish had probably been thinking of it all day as we were talking around him. That was a shocking and beautiful moment for all of us.

It reminded me of a situation I experienced years earlier with my father-in-law, who also had dementia. He always had tremendous respect for his oldest brother, Mendel; both were Auschwitz survivors. Uncle Mendel was dying of cancer, but was still very alert. He asked his children to bring him to visit his brother, who was very sick and completely non-verbal.

Uncle Mendel was begging my father-in-law to recognize him; it was heartbreaking for all of us to see.

"Please tell me you know I'm here," Uncle Mendel begged.

But my father-in-law remained silent.

Two days later, however, my father-in-law spoke.

"My brother Mendel was here," he whispered.

He probably had it stored in his mind, and without any prompting, it came out. It was an amazing and eye-opening moment.

***

There are certain songs that our family sang every week on the Sabbath. There was one in particular—*Baruch Kel Elyon*—that Moish liked very much.

In March of 2012, I was singing with some of my friends and my granddaughter, when Moish's Uncle Yossi came to visit. After World War II, in which Moish's grandparents were killed, Uncle Yossi lived with Moish's parents, his brother, and his sister-in-law. Moish had a special attachment to him partially because they lived in the same house when Moish was young.

Now that Uncle Yossi saw how sick his nephew was, he wanted to take care of him—he used to come over on Saturday afternoons. He prayed at the synagogue across the street from us, and came to visit us after prayers.

On one particular Saturday, when Uncle Yossi came by, Moish was a bit on the sad side. I suggested to Uncle Yossi that perhaps he could sing *Baruch Kel Elyon*, the song Moish loved.

Uncle Yossi began to sing with a tremendous amount of emotion and heart—but he did much more than that. He delicately stood Moish up and began to dance with him. I could see in Moish's face how happy this made him—it was the power of music, and the power of somebody familiar from years back, and the amazing power of touch.

***

Along this difficult journey, G-d has sent me a few "angels" along the way. One of the most memorable was a young medical student named Lauren, who came to visit us when Moish was in the hospital under Dr. Gold's supervision. We spent a lot of time together during the week, and she was helpful because she could relay messages to the doctor, who I wasn't able to get hold of otherwise.

Beyond that, it was helpful to have a young, optimistic medical person to talk to; she was able to tell me what she thought was going to happen. Lauren was very bright and full of information.

Not all my angels were to be found in the hospital, however. One of them I encountered, in all places, at Chase Bank.

This woman saw me texting, and asked me if I paid my bills online.

"I have no clue how to do that," I laughed.

"Sit down," she told me. "I'm going to show you how to pay your bills online."

This amazing woman sat there with me like she had all the time in the world. She didn't know me from a hole in the wall, but she taught me everything I needed to know. I went home right away and paid my bills so I wouldn't forget; this woman saved me an incredible amount of time.

I went back to Chase a few times to thank her, but I never saw her again. It's almost like she stopped working there, and that G-d sent her to teach me this little trick. Looking back, it seems very minor, but considering all the stress I had in my life, it felt like a very big gift indeed!

***

Needless to say, it became hard for me to "get away" from the chaos of my daily life. Occasionally I was able to sneak away for a few hours at a time, but for the most part I spent my weekends with Moish. Most of the time we stayed at home, but occasionally we went away, although it was becoming increasingly difficult to take Moish anywhere new. It put him out of sorts, which made the trip unpleasant for him and for me.

I had one son who lived in Brooklyn; we often ate lunch together on Shabbos. I enjoyed this very much, but I had other kids who I wanted to see as well. On top of that I was working at HASC, so I didn't have many opportunities to see them. I really wanted to see my other kids, but was tortured over whether it was fair for me to leave Moish on the weekends.

When I became conflicted, I called my cousin David, who always encouraged me.

"It's okay, you can do this," he said. "Get in that car and go."

On the rare occasions that I did go away, I would sit down and explain the situation to Moish.

"I'm going to go away," I would tell him. "It's Friday today, and I'm going to come back tomorrow night."

I never waited until Sunday—I always came home as soon as the sun went down on Saturday. When I told Moish I was going to visit the kids, he seemed to understand what I was saying.

One day when I was telling him my plans, he looked right at me and said, very quietly, "Please come back."

He wasn't telling me not to go—he just wanted me to reassure him that I would come back after my trip.

"Of course I'm coming back," I said. "I'm only going to visit the kids; I'll be back tomorrow night."

He seemed okay with that—although, to be honest, I wasn't one-hundred percent sure he wasn't really telling me not to go at all. But I was pretty sure, because he wasn't crying or agitated when he said it. He said it very calmly.

When I got in the car I started crying. I called David, who told me to keep driving. I had a wonderful visit with my son; it was exactly what I needed. For my own sanity, I needed to get away every so often.

Unfortunately, with every passing year, leaving Moish became more stressful. I had a horrible, nagging voice in the back of my head: "You don't know how much longer Moish is going to live. What if you leave and something happens? How will you forgive yourself?"

I felt guilty because Moish understood that I was leaving. I've heard people refer to this as "Jewish guilt," but I think that everybody has a bit of that kind of guilt when it comes to their own family.

***

Throughout my life, I was the kind of person who had a few really close friends, as opposed to dozens of superficial friends. I'm a very intense person, so when I like somebody, I *really* like them. As Moish got more and more sick, I found myself returning to my roots, contacting friends from "my old life." I reached out to people who knew me before I got married—they gave me a lot of comfort, because we could talk about "the old days," and not just about my life with Moish.

There was a woman named Bonnie I met when I was in high school in Baltimore. She was thirteen years older than me and had a completely different lifestyle than I did, but we bonded anyway. She became like a surrogate mother to me.

Bonnie had a house full of kids, which was my dream, so I spent as much time as I could at her house. I helped her with her kids, and we grew extremely close over the years. At some point, sadly, we lost track of each other. I moved away to Israel, and Bonnie moved away as well.

When Moish got sick, however, I felt a desperate need to reach out to Bonnie. At first I couldn't find her address, but with the help of my children and the Internet, I ultimately tracked her down and reconnected with her. Once we reconnected, it was like no time had passed, and we've remained close ever since.

Having a sick husband changed me, and my family, in numerous ways. It made me more introspective and more determined to enjoy every moment I spent with my loved ones. Moish was having trouble navigating through life, so I steeled myself the best I could, because deep down I knew that this was only the beginning.

I reached a point where I felt more like Hennie Bak—my maiden name—than Hennie Friedman. The sicker Moish got, the more I felt like the woman I was before I got married.

***

Although I was dealing with Moish's illness, it didn't mean that we were immune to other challenges. In 2013 I was tested further when one of my children went through a very difficult personal situation. In a strange way I was glad that Moish had no clue. I don't think he would have handled it well.

At this time I began to get a little bit angry with G-d.

"You gave me a sick husband, and I'm dealing with that," I cried and begged to G-d. "But now you're pushing it. This is more than I can bear."

I need my children to be well. Over the next few years things got better, and life was good to me once again.

One thing I realized during this ordeal was that even though we cry and pray for important things, we can still ask G-d for menial things. Sometimes I had trouble saying morning prayers, but I began feeling content having conversations in my head or saying the words out loud. I made a conscious effort to think about G-d all day long.

In the morning, I'd say, "G-d, I really need a parking spot... could you get me one?" I would keep this sort of conversation up for the entire day. It kept me focused, and reminded me that G-d was always with me.

When Moish and I came back from our trip to Israel in 2006, I noticed that I got better with acts of everyday kindness, but worse with routine prayers. I forgave myself for this, and I hope G-d forgave me too.

I did many things I would never have done if Moish hadn't gotten sick... but they were sometimes things I had little control over. I continued every day to work on improving myself.

CHAPTER 10

One Sunday, I took the train to Baltimore to visit a friend, Laurie, whom I had been close to since high school. She was an energetic, upbeat, amazing person, and I was crushed to learn that she was dying of cancer.

Laurie was always outstanding, but when she got cancer, she rose a step above. Instead of falling apart, like so many people do, the cancer motivated her, and she became an inspirational speaker. Any time she had a drop of energy, she was doing something special for somebody else.

The last time I visited her, which was weeks before she died, I told her I had a confession to make.

"What's your confession?" she asked.

A few years earlier, Laurie had heard what was going on with Moish, and on a trip into New York she wanted to visit him.

Laurie didn't realize how sick Moish truly was, so she called and asked if she could see him—in ten minutes!

I was in the house at the time, and I told Moish, "I'm leaving the house for a while." I wasn't in the mood to be cheerful, even for someone I loved.

I left the house as quickly as I could, because I couldn't face her. As it turned out, when she arrived Moish wasn't there either because he had no memory of their conversation, so he went out for a bit.

I was sorry that I couldn't face Laurie, or make sure that Moish could see her.

I regretted my behavior. I felt guilty, because Moish really liked her. It was a very selfish moment, but I simply wasn't able to cope with visitors at that time.

Laurie told me that she was happy that I told her and that I could get it off my chest. I loved her for understanding.

***

Not all of the books I read were specifically about dementia. I have always liked to read heroic and uplifting books, no matter the subject. One of my favorite authors was Cathy Glass, a foster parent to over one hundred kids who wrote about twenty books on the subject. I read every single one of them, and then sent her an email telling her how much she inspired me.

It didn't matter who they were or what their background was—Jewish or not, religious or irreligious—I was drawn to authors who gallantly pushed through difficulties. I had always loved reading those types of books, but now I appreciated them on an entirely new level.

***

In the summer of 2014, Moish began having some serious skin issues—undoubtedly from his wheelchair. At first I thought it was from being in bed all day, but ultimately, I pegged his wheelchair as the culprit.

Moish was getting out a lot in his wheelchair. Norma picked him up in the morning and took him to the Senior Center, and they often didn't return until two o'clock in the afternoon. Moish spent the entire time sitting in his wheelchair, which wasn't custom-made, although it did have a special cushion.

Moish's skin looked so terrible that I hired a wound-care specialist to make a home visit to help us heal his skin. Soon after that, Moish ended up in the hospital with pneumonia. He was on a regular mattress, and the nurses weren't great at moving or turning him. But his skin still healed, and that's when I realized it was the wheelchair that was causing his issues, not the bed.

The way Moish was sitting in the wheelchair was causing breakdowns in the skin near the bottom of his spine. I started telling Norma to limit the amount of time Moish spent in his wheelchair. He went to the Senior Center less often, and when he returned home with Norma, she got him out of the chair as soon as possible.

Eventually, we bought Moish a custom wheelchair that fit his body exactly—but even in a custom model, it was still worse for his skin than being in the bed. My son-in-law gave us an expensive hospital mattress that constantly circulated air. It was truly a godsend.

Sitting is harder on a body than lying down. As grateful as I was for the healing that the wound specialist provided to Moish, it was the realization that it was the wheelchair causing his sores, rather than the bed, that made all the difference.

***

Every so often, Moish would reveal a rare and beautiful sense of humor. Some of his funniest moments were reserved for his aides, each of whom had their own terrific sense of humor. One day one of Moish's aides, Norma, dyed her wig a bright, iridescent blue, which Moish thought was fantastic.

"You're crazy," he told her, and Norma laughed right along with him. Her reaction was beautiful to watch—she could have been angry with him or gotten hurt feelings, but instead she was able to laugh at herself. She was able to find humor in the little things that Moish did or said, and this made his life and my life so much easier.

Another day he was taking a walk in his wheelchair with Norma. Moish was in a very good mood, and in a rare moment of clarity, he flipped himself around and loudly exclaimed, "Oh my goodness, you're not my wife!"

Norma laughed her head off along with Moish—it was such a great moment for her to be part of. It was these kinds of incidents where Norma and I had a choice to make—if we couldn't laugh about it, we would have no choice but to cry.

***

One of the hardest things for me to witness was when Moish was no longer able to eat with his mouth, but instead was forced to use a feeding tube.

It started out with Moish having pneumonia—but not the "normal" kind where a cold turns into pneumonia. There is another kind called aspiration pneumonia, which you can get when you're not eating and have reflux. Somebody like Moish, who is fed through a tube, can get pneumonia when food from their feeding tube comes up and goes into the wrong place.

I didn't know much about that at the time; I only knew that Moish was aspirating, and a lot of times he would cough during his feedings. This made Moish very upset, and sometimes he would get so agitated that he'd begin turning purple. I kept trying different things—feeding him slower, or using a bolus feeding tube, in which you put all of the food in an open syringe and it slowly goes down into the G-tube.

At the beginning, I wanted to do a combination of tube feeding and regular feeding. It was vital that Moish got the right amount of nutrition, but I wanted him to get some enjoyment out of the actual food as well.

Unfortunately, Moish was coughing so much that he wasn't getting nutrition *or* enjoyment. I knew that if I could give him a can or two of formula, he would be fine.

I had a close friend, Esther, who had a grandchild with a feeding tube; she liked to prepare a huge pot of chicken and vegetables, which she would then blend up. She froze this into plastic bags with single-sized portions. My friend stocked my entire freezer with these meals; I could take one bag out in the morning and lunch would be ready to go.

Moish had good feeding sessions and bad feeding sessions; we took our cues from him. It went from twenty percent tube feeding, to fifty percent tube feeding, to ninety-nine percent tube feeding. Once in a blue moon Norma would feed him applesauce with thickit. If she felt he was thirsty, she would give him a little bit of thickened water by mouth.

Sometimes we would cheat, just to give him the pleasure of eating something like ice cream, which Moish wasn't supposed to have. In general, thin foods weren't as good as thick foods like Jell-O. But sometimes I just wanted Moish to experience that pleasure. When we gave him ice cream, he would laugh, so we knew he was enjoying it. Every time he laughed, I felt guilty, thinking I should do it more often.

One day I prepared a pot of pureed vegetable soup; I gave it to my aide to feed to Moish.

Moish tasted it and said, "Thank G-d!" which was his way of saying he was finally tasting some home-cooked food.

I took my cues from Norma; she was with Moish all day, so she knew when he was having a day that he could eat, and when he wasn't.

Watching Moish eat, I felt the same way I felt at work when a child was unable to eat a food they once loved; it was sad because they could still *smell* the food.

Most of all, I felt sad for Moish because he was being denied one of the great pleasures of life—being able to enjoy good food.

***

By the summer of 2014, I had become depressed because I didn't know if Moish knew me anymore. It was extremely hard for me when he lost his verbal communication—although it was even worse when he partially lost his ability to smile. His smile had always been his signature, and it threw me for a loop when it was gone.

Moish had a lot of different facial expressions. For instance, he would pucker his lips to show me he wanted to kiss me, or he'd give me a surprised or loving look.

By that terrible summer, the only thing Moish was capable of doing, expression-wise, was to raise his eyebrows to let me know he had heard me. Outside of that, I hadn't received much verbal or non-verbal communication for months.

One of the nurses I spoke to suggested I give Moish an antidepressant. At first this made me angry, because all I could think about were the potential side effects. Once I thought about it, however, I began to consider it but decided against it. I was afraid to start Moish on a new medication when things were stable, although I was always on the lookout for anything that would make things better for him.

***

Moish and I met Yocheved Weingott in 1985 when we lived in Israel. At the time she was five years old. There was something extremely special about Yocheved. When we moved back to New York, she and I stayed in touch. As she got older, Yocheved moved back and forth between Israel and America. She was destined to be part of my life. I once ran into her when she was seventeen and looking for an apartment in New York. All she had was her luggage, so I grabbed it, threw it in my car, and insisted that she move in with me for a few months. We have remained close ever since.

Shortly after Moish became ill, Yocheved visited us for the weekend. Other than my immediate family, she was one of the few people I felt comfortable having at our home overnight. Yocheved was warm, loving, non-judgmental, and easygoing. I needed somebody like her because with Moish, I never knew what was going to happen. The last thing I needed was to worry about what my company was going to see.

With Yocheved, I could be myself—and, more importantly, I could do whatever I wanted and not worry about her reaction. I was just happy to have her in my house.

On this particular Shabbos, near dinnertime on Saturday, I told Yocheved that I was going downstairs for a moment. We generally have one big meal on the Sabbath at lunchtime, followed by a smaller meal toward evening.

On this occasion, I told Yocheved, "Why don't you stay with Moish. I'll go downstairs and prepare the meal, and we'll eat together."

Five minutes later, she came running down the steps; I thought for a moment that something was wrong.

"You're not going to believe this," Yocheved said.

She told me that while she was alone with Moish, he asked her, "Where is she?"

"You mean Hennie?" Yocheved asked.

Moish wanted me back in the room with him.

"You go upstairs to your husband," Yocheved insisted. "I'll prepare the food."

That was during a time when Moish wasn't communicating much, so to have him say something like that was a true gift to me. The moment was made better because Yocheved was the person who got to tell me that Moish was asking for me. I didn't think he was capable of that. Those moments, so few and far between, were extremely special to me.

***

Sometimes many weeks went by at once where Moish showed very little sign of recognition or understanding. One day I was trying to reposition Moish, even though I didn't have the physical strength that some of my aides had. Despite my best efforts to make Moish comfortable, he looked upset. He clearly wanted to tell me something, but didn't have the words.

Finally, in a big, loud, booming voice—his *old* voice— Moish yelled, "HENNIE!"

I hadn't heard him speak my name for several months, and hearing my name come from his mouth was music to my ears; it kept me going for the next several weeks.

***

Near the end of 2014, I saw a creative wedding proposal online—it was one of those flash mobs that was so popular at the time.

In the video, the groom had flown his family in from out of town. People were laughing and crying, and the entire group of people was dancing. I was astounded by the beauty and emotion of it all.

After I watched it—several times—I cried because I so badly wanted to show it to Moish, but I knew he wouldn't get anything out of it. I couldn't share things like that with him anymore, because he couldn't absorb what I was showing him.

It wasn't just online wedding proposal flash mobs that made me cry—in truth, almost anything made me cry when I was in a certain state of mind.

One thing that made me sad was that I didn't feel like I could write anymore, because I didn't feel like I had anything inspiring left to say.

Pinky wisely told me that people don't always want to be inspired; sometimes they want to hear things as they really are, even if those things are difficult. People don't always want to feel like somebody else is a superman or a superwoman. They want you to "say it like it is."

I decided that Pinky was probably right. I hadn't written a word for months, even though it was my dream one day to lecture across the world about my personal experience as a caretaker for somebody with Lewy Body Dementia. I wanted to spread the message that nobody really understands how much people with dementia process and hear. There's a lot of guesswork involved, and Moish often shocked me—in a good way—with the things he said and did.

I feel down on a lot of days, and I look at my beautiful husband, who is still well-groomed most of the time, and wish he could take me in his arms and comfort me. Sadly, it doesn't look like that is ever going to happen, so I just need to come to terms with it.

***

For most of the time since we returned from Israel in 1988, I worked as a nurse for HASC, but for a period of three years, I left the school and worked in several HASC group homes with young adults.

I was their nurse, and because I went back frequently to visit, I grew to know and love some of the young adults who lived there. Although I hadn't worked at that job for many years, I did remember one Chassidic young man who was high functioning; he used to take the bus to go say morning prayers with his father, who was a rabbi. This young man had been specifically trained to take the bus by the people at the group home.

Several years later, I made a financial decision to give up my car; I reasoned that if I did this, I would have more money to buy gifts for my grandchildren. Buying presents for my grandchildren was my favorite thing in the world, and it bothered me that I was strapped for cash and didn't have much money to do that. Between the insurance, the lease, the gas, and the insurance, the car became one of my biggest expenses.

It was a tossup—Legos for the grandkids or a car for me. I ultimately got rid of the car because I didn't travel much; the only place I drove the car was to work, which wasn't far at all. On the occasions that I ventured out to Far Rockaway to visit my children, Zevi, who lived a few blocks away from me, gladly lent me his car.

For two years I used public transportation, which wasn't a big deal because the bus ran close by our house. I took the same bus to work every morning, and was pleased to see the Chassidic young man from the group home was still taking the bus to go and say prayers with his father.

This young man had a constant cough, the type that was from allergies as opposed to sickness. Sometimes he struggled and forgot to cover his mouth when he coughed. People were disgusted by his behavior.

There were always the same passengers with us on the bus, and I could see many of them moving away from him. Some of them made nasty comments, which bothered me.

After observing this for a few days, I couldn't take their behavior anymore. One morning after the young man had gotten off the bus, I turned to one particularly nasty man and said, "You know that man who just got off the bus?"

"Yes," he said.

"He might be an adult," I explained, "but he's challenged mentally, and he can't help himself."

The nasty man looked genuinely upset.

"I'm sorry," he said. "I didn't mean to offend you."

"You didn't offend me," I said to him. "But that man has feelings, and the way you talk to him is very hurtful. It's not something he has control over, so you need to be aware."

The nasty man and some of the others listened to what I had to say, although I was worried they were going to tell me off. They didn't get in my face, but the whole interaction made me wonder who said what to Moish when he took the bus.

Thinking about the Chassidic young man, there was an "adult" who was, sometimes, no different than a scared little boy. Furthermore, most people on that bus didn't know that, in general, Chassidic men don't strike up friendly conversations with women who are not their spouses. They generally don't socialize with women, except their immediate family members. Often the women sit at one table and the men sit at another.

Even so, every time he saw me he got excited. This young man looked normal, and wore normal-looking clothes; it was just his behavior that bothered people.

If I hadn't been going through a similar situation with Moish, I'm not sure I would have confronted the other passengers. I would have been angry, but most likely I would have been *quietly* angry.

***

There were a handful of people who Moish knew well in high school, people he spent a tremendous amount of time with. As young married couples, we went out together occasionally. Once or twice a year we'd get together for dinner during the holidays.

Some of those people made an effort to visit Moish when he was sick, which must have been hard on them emotionally. I was amazed that they seemed to have stronger feelings for Moish than many of the people we saw every day.

They were people who bonded with Moish through many, many years when they were very young. It was beautiful to see how emotional they were, and how happy they made Moish when they came over to visit. It meant so much to him because they really were his closest friends. Their friendship was something he could claim for himself.

Even though we used to get together as couples, their strong relationship was with Moish and his former classmates. I tried my hardest to stay in the background so that Moish could celebrate his own friendship with them. It was very special for him, and it was equally special for me to watch.

There were other people who simply couldn't bring themselves to visit Moish in his sick condition, and although I understood, it was still hurtful on some level.

It came to a point where I didn't want anybody to see Moish except those few people who had been in touch with him throughout his illness. I felt comfortable with those who were able to gracefully handle the deterioration, the hallucinations, and the loss of dignity. I only wanted people to visit if they could see through all of that to what a beautiful person Moish still was.

There was one man in particular who came over nearly every single Saturday. He was as dedicated to Moish as anybody I've ever met. I felt that if people didn't see Moish in the earlier stages of the disease when he was more alert, perhaps now wasn't the best time to come. He wasn't looking great, and drooling occasionally. It was great for Moish to see faces he still recognized to some degree.

***

Years ago, Malkie gave me a journal, and after that, Ruchi gave me the same one. On the cover it said:

It's not about waiting for the storm to pass. It's about learning to dance in the rain.

I first saw this saying on somebody's desk at work; I thought it was a brilliant and applicable saying to my life. First, I adore the rain, and love to walk around in it. It can be the windiest, stormiest day, where everybody is complaining about the weather, and I'm as happy as a lark, so "dancing in the rain" had a special meaning to me.

I remember years earlier when Moish came home after I'd had an abnormally hectic day.

"How was your day," he asked.

"My day?" I said. "I sat in a bubble bath eating bon-bons; my day was awesome!"

Moish said, "You know that's not why we're here. We face challenges… to grow. Every day has challenges, and our job is to face those challenges and learn from them."

At the time, those words went in one of my ears and out the other; I simply wouldn't listen to him. But when Moish got sick he said the same thing in such a dignified manner that I knew he really believed his words.

The saying was a reflection of what Moish felt. Another person who was like that was my grandfather, my mother's father. He was very stoic. When my mother lost her oldest child, Pinky, my grandfather told her, "On Sabbath, you have to be happy. You have to sing… you can't cry."

She would think, "What a terribly cruel thing to say," but when his own wife passed away, my grandfather sat at the table and sang all the songs. In other words, he was *not* a hypocrite; when you see somebody who is actually sincere in their beliefs, it's easier to accept. That's how I felt about Moish.

CHAPTER 11

In 2015, Moish kept getting terrible abscesses on various parts of his body. I treated them and drained them, and then prepared dressings to help them heal. One particular abscess looked so awful that my health aide and I decided to take Moish to the emergency room. We wheeled him the several blocks there since it was so difficult to get him into a car.

The hospital checked Moish out and released him, but the next day I received a call from the hospital. The culture they took on the abscess came back positive for MSRA, a type of resistant staph infection that required intravenous antibiotics. That was the diagnosis I had expected; if I hadn't, I wouldn't have taken him to the hospital in the first place.

I left work as soon as I was able, and brought Moish back to the hospital. They treated him for several days with Vancomycin, which was administered through a peripherally inserted central catheter, otherwise known as a Picc line. The problem was that every day that Moish took the medication, his breathing became worse. After a few days, I was told I could bring Moish home as long as I continued to give him his medication through the Picc line for another two weeks; I had to have somebody come in and teach me how to run the Picc line, even though I was a nurse. They didn't think that his breathing issues had anything to do with the medication.

One or two days into being at home, I thought that Moish was dying. He literally couldn't breathe, and I could hear him gasping all the way down the hall.

I began to cry.

"This is the end," I told myself. "We're done."

Then I had a thought. Maybe it really was the medication that was affecting his breathing. When I called the doctor, he told me that wasn't a typical side effect of the medicine.

I asked him to stop the medication anyway, and he agreed to give me an oral medication instead. Once he stopped the Picc line, Moish's breathing improved every day.

Sometimes I felt that the doctors didn't believe me—but I stubbornly proceeded to do what I believed to be in Moish's best interest.

***

Bringing Moish to the hospital brought about an unforeseen complication—once a patient was admitted to the hospital, their health aides were no longer able to come via the agency. Therefore we had the choice either to stay at the hospital, or to pay privately for health aides.

We elected to do both, but the hospital claimed that Moish no longer belonged at home because he was so sick. They wanted to transfer him to a nursing home, which was something that Moish and I had discussed earlier in his sickness. I reassured Moish that putting him in a nursing home was not an option, and that I would never do so willingly.

My advocate, Malka Fass, and Zevi fought for me for three days on this issue… and won! We were allowed to bring Moish home, and my aides were reinstated.

I told Zevi that from now on, unless there was an immediate life and death situation, we were *not* taking Moish to the hospital. Even if we had to call an ambulance and go to the emergency room, we could still refuse to get admitted to the hospital.

This added a lot of stress to my life, as I often feared that my aides would have to call an ambulance, and that Moish would be transported to the hospital. Obviously, if I wasn't there I couldn't tell them not to call an ambulance if they felt they must.

***

Moish got to the point where he could no longer sit in his standard wheelchair. He could hold his head up in the wheelchair for a period of time, but after awhile, especially when he was tired, his head would start to lean to the left side. This was terribly uncomfortable for Moish. We tried to remedy this situation with a cervical collar, but it was unsuccessful. I knew it was time to measure Moish for a custom-made wheelchair.

I contacted a wheelchair expert named Gary, who specialized in making custom-made wheelchairs; he constructed wheelchairs for several of the kids at HASC. He told me that as far as a head support, anything I bought that would really work would be cumbersome and uncomfortable for Moish. So we had Gary construct a custom-built wheelchair, and we had to allow Moish to tilt his head to the side. We couldn't remedy that. Part of Lewy Body is some curvature of the spine, which affected Moish's posture, as well as his ability to keep his head up.

Moish's new wheelchair was the best investment we ever made. It allowed Norma to take Moish on long walks when I was at work. She often brought him to my kids' houses on Shabbos and *Yom Tov*, which was great for all of us.

The first time that Norma took Moish out in his new chair, Moish said to her, twice, "THANK you so much!"

Norma was overcome with emotion, and was grateful to make Moish so happy. Moish hadn't spoken in weeks, but he still managed to thank Norma. He wanted to be sure that she heard him, so he repeated himself just in case. Norma then walked with Moish to visit my daughter Ruchi, to tell her what happened—and they both cried. It was truly unbelievable.

***

My mother passed away in the summer of 2015. It was a sad occasion, of course, but we were grateful that she lived a full, vibrant life, and welcomed her Creator at the age of 91. Like many daughters before me, I felt a fair amount of guilt at her passing—guilt that I didn't do enough for her, guilt that I didn't take care of her the way I should have. The truth was, I was so overwhelmed and busy taking care of Moish, I hoped that my mother understood and was able to forgive me.

Along with my guilt, I felt a small measure of relief. My mother suffered in her last few months, and I believed that she was now at peace. Once she passed, I wanted to move to Far Rockaway to be closer to several of my kids. Thankfully, my home health aides agreed to stay with me even though two of them lived in Brooklyn. I felt that moving would make things better for Moish, for me, and hopefully for our children as well. I never would have moved while my mother was living in Brooklyn; she lived a five-minute drive from my home, and we spent a great deal of time together.

For several years, I felt that life would be easier if we moved out of our beloved home in Brooklyn. It wasn't practical for us to have a four-story house, and although I put a special wheelchair lift at the bottom of the stairs, it was still difficult going up and down.

Although we made many beautiful memories in our home, the last few years were fraught with difficulties and bittersweet moments. My kids, especially the younger ones, had a strong bond with the house they grew up in, but they understood that it was time for me to move into a condominium in the Five Towns.

Downsizing was a huge relief to me. There's a Jewish expression that says, "The more possessions one acquires, the more worries." I found this to be an accurate statement for me, especially since I was responsible for anything and everything that needed to be fixed. Every leak, crack, and plumbing issue was my job, and I was happy to move to smaller quarters. I relished not having to take the garbage to the curb, and not having to hire someone to shovel the snow.

The best part of the condominium was the porch, which had a clear view of the beach. It was a gift to watch the sun set over the serene waters. I relished the view of the beach and of the neighborhood.

I had wanted to move for a long time, but felt that it would not have worked when Moish was still coherent and sociable. The number of visitors had dwindled, and there was little verbal communication between me and Moish, so I began to feel lonely on the weekends. When my mother passed away, it was just a matter of time before I decided to sell my house.

Once I made up my mind, the entire packing and moving process took about six months. I felt that was impressive, considering how much we had accumulated over the thirty years we lived there. I knew that I had to choose carefully, as we were moving into a lovely but relatively small two-bedroom condominium.

On moving day, my kids came to help me, and within a day or two, we had a functioning apartment. I was happy to give away many things that we no longer needed. I gave away almost all of my silver and jewelry to my children and grandchildren, which gave me great pleasure. I was just as happy wearing costume jewelry, and now I didn't have to worry about losing something valuable or sentimental. My books and pictures were my greatest treasures. I gave away many books to family friends and to the synagogue where we prayed.

I had so many photo albums that I decided to temporarily store them in my daughter's attic. Over time, I took apart the albums and sorted the pictures into boxes—the 1980s, the 1990s, and so on. Instead of countless albums, I consolidated my pictures into several large boxes that fit into my closet, which was a very positive experience.

We moved in October of 2016, and although I was ecstatic to move, Moish didn't deal well with the change. Zevi drove Moish to Far Rockaway, and Moish vomited all over the car and all over himself. Zevi didn't want to tell me, and I wondered why it took them so long to arrive. Moish couldn't verbally express his fears and concerns, which made things extremely difficult for him. Despite my reassurance, Moish acted very sad, and I worried that he thought I might be placing him in a nursing home, or abandoning him in some manner.

Every day I reassured Moish that this was a move for both of us, and that all of his aides would remain the same. I was home a lot because of the holidays, which made things easier for Moish, but it took several weeks until he seemed content and relaxed in our new home. It brought both of us immeasurable joy to see so many more of our kids on a regular basis. Zevi and his family frequently came to visit us over the weekends, and the out-of-towners came in whenever possible.

***

In 2017, shortly after New Year's, Moish had a terrible seizure just after midnight. I had to administer two doses of Diastat before his seizures abated. At 6:00 a.m., Moish had another seizure, and I was forced to use my last dose of Diastat. Even though I had vowed to avoid hospitals, I was in a panic at the thought of Moish having another seizure and having no more medication. I asked my cousin Dr. Leb to call in more Diastat to the local pharmacy. I also remembered that Klonopin lowered the threshold for seizures, so I gave Moish some Klonopin and thanked *Hashem* for my nursing experience and for Dr. Leb. I then took the day off from work to stay with Moish.

In February, it seemed that Moish lost his beautiful smile. Rarely did his face light up, and rarely did he seem to recognize me. Although there were definitely moments when his eyes showed their special sparkle, most of the time he did not show recognition. Sadly, there was no way to know either way. At times, conversing with him was difficult. My children bought us the large-size hospital bed with the mattress that circulated the air, so Moish and I were able to lay next to each other and listen to music, or watch television, or simply hold hands. This brought me a great deal of comfort, and I prayed that Moish felt the same way.

***

I read a beautiful story that I have repeated to several people. There was a man waiting on line at the post office. He was impatient, and desperately wanted the line to move faster.

"I don't know if I can wait any longer," he said. "I need to get to the nursing home to see my wife."

"You visit her every day?" a second man asked.

"Yes," the man said. "I go every day at the exact same time before lunch."

"Does your wife wait for you?" the second man asked.

"She doesn't wait," the man said. "In fact, she has no idea who I am."

"Maybe you don't have to go every day," the second man said.

"My wife may not know who I am," the man said. "But I still know who she is."

This story struck a chord with me. It reminded me that it's not always about *getting* something. I wanted to give as much as possible to the man I committed to spend my life with more than forty years ago—the man who also happens to be my best friend.

***

When Moish suffered some additional medical issues in 2017, I placed him on home hospice with MJHS for a few months. He improved so much that after several weeks, we took him off hospice for an entire year!

When Moish once again faced difficult medical issues, hospice reevaluated him and started once again. Although several people told me that hospice gives up on the patient and only makes them comfortable, I found that to be completely false. They provided us with all of the equipment we needed such as oxygen and a nebulizer with medication. There was someone available to speak to 24/7, which was useful and amazing. A doctor came periodically and was able to be consulted for emergencies. A nurse came once a week. They prescribed antibiotics as needed, and were open to all the suggestions and questions that I asked. I found hospice to be a gift that gave me a tremendous amount of peace of mind.

***

In the spring of 2017, Pinky came over on Purim with a group of his friends. Purim is the joyous holiday that celebrates the defeat of Haman's plot to massacre the Jews, as recorded in the book of Esther the Queen. Pinky's friends came dressed in costumes, surrounded Moish's bed, and pulled out their guitars. The music and singing were absolutely beautiful. Moish was overcome with emotion, and tears began running down his face. It had been a long time since we had witnessed such a strong level of emotion from Moish. He was listening and appreciating the music and the holiday spirit, a day that is joyous for the Jewish people.

I often attempted to make Moish comfortable in his bed, but as hard as I tried, I never did as professional a job as my health aides. I was blown away by their skills. I did not possess their physical strength. One day Kim walked in and Moish needed to be adjusted in his bed. He took one look at Kim and said "Thank G-d!" I knew that she could make him so much more comfortable than I could, and he was so grateful. My jobs included providing the supplies, preparing the meds, resolving medical issues, and otherwise being a wife.

***

One morning on my drive in to Brooklyn, my aide Guylene called me. It was still quite early so I knew there must be a problem, and there was—Moish's g-tube was clogged, and no food was passing through. I wasn't far away, so I returned home and replaced the g-tube. I always tried to keep a spare tube in case of emergency. It worried me that had I been out of town, this small issue might have turned into a fiasco, requiring a trip to the hospital. That fear kept me from traveling for several months, which saddened me because I wanted to be able to visit my kids who lived in Florida and Chicago. I started to feel distanced from them to the point that I said, "Enough is enough."

I needed to take a chance and take some short vacations in order to spend quality time with my kids and grandkids. I was so happy that I could go, as well as grateful that there were no emergencies in New York.

I tried my best to be there for Moish, but there were times when I knew that the right thing to do might be to go away for a bit. It kept me in better spirits, and less depressed; I felt that if I never left, I jeopardized the special relationships that I treasured with family and close friends. It was a hard call to make. I tried to take one day at a time, since every day brought new challenges and concerns, as well as blessings.

I pray to have the physical and mental health to keep going and to stay upbeat. When Moish and I received the official diagnosis of Lewy Body Dementia in 2008, I had already known for several years that Moish had a serious illness. The neurologist told me then that that the average life span from diagnosis is six to eight years.

We have far surpassed those years. I sometimes wonder whether or not that's a good thing. I do know one thing, and that is that I promised Moish that I would take care of him to the best of my ability, and to keep him pain-free as much as possible.

As for the rest of it, I leave it all in G-d's hands.

ABOUT THE AUTHOR

Hennie Friedman lives in Far Rockaway, New York. She can be reached at henniefriedman1@gmail.com.

www.ingramcontent.com/pod-product-compliance
Lightning Source LLC
Chambersburg PA
CBHW020317290526
45785CB00007B/2827